The Autistic Author and Animator

Library and Archives Canada Cataloguing in Publication

Walmsley, Janet, 1955-, author
    The autistic author and animator : a mother's view of a daughter's
triumph / Janet Walmsley.

Issued in print and electronic formats.
ISBN 978-1-77141-105-9 (pbk.).--ISBN 978-1-77141-106-6 (html)

    1. Walmsley, Jenny. 2. Autistic people--Biography. 3. Authors--
Biography. 4. Animators--Biography. 5. Walmsley, Janet, 1955-.
6. Mothers of autistic children--Biography. I. Title.

HQ773.8.W25 2015   618.92'858820092   C2015-901232-5
                                                C2015-901233-3

The Autistic Author and Animator

A Mother's View of a Daughter's Triumph

Janet Walmsley

Book Cover Design: Trista Baldwin
Cover photographer: Amanda Waschuk
Editor: Nina Shoroplova
Assistant Editor: Sue Kehoe
Production Editor: Jennifer Kaleta
Typeset: Greg Salisbury
Portrait Photographer: Tobyn Ross of Tobyn Ross Photography

For my daughter, Jenny Story. You are a pillar of strength. For your love, courage, kindness, and genuine spirit. You are an inspiration to me and a role model to so many others.

Testimonials

"Janet writes with freshness, truth, and love. That is how she is able to bring us along to share her experiences in raising her remarkable daughter Jenny."
Betty Watson, Author of *On a Day in Brandon Manitoba 9/9/99* and *What Can Jordyn Do*

"With a deep bond of love, irrepressible optimism and unquenchable determination, Janet and Jenny together gain strength from every challenge they face. A warm, joy-filled book that teaches us to never give up, and to always be proud of who we are and the unique gifts we have to share."
Margaret Hudson, Respite Care Coordinator

"Janet Walmsley writes like she is sitting having coffee at the kitchen table sharing with a dear friend about her daughter Jenny's story. A triumphant journey. I always knew and said with confidence, 'Jenny will fly.'"
Gail Cunningham, ECE Supervisor and Owner of Brer Rabbit Day Care

Acknowledgements

I would like to lovingly thank, number one, my daughter Jenny for letting me expose her life out in the open.

I lovingly thank my son Christopher and my husband Travis for being so supportive and cheering me on in writing this book. Most of all your love, genuine care, support, and cheering on Jenny each and every day of her life. I love you both so much.

I gratefully thank all the professionals on our "Dream Team" who went above and beyond with their time and support for Jenny—Darlene Wolsey, Lisa Coley Donahue, Fran Wood, Dr. Waida, and Dr. Bruce Pipher.

To Gail, Deb, Shelley, Teresa, and the rest of the staff at Brer Rabbit Day Care, words cannot express enough our thanks, gratitude, and love for your care and love of Jenny. You were rocks to both Jenny and me.

Our love and thanks to Margaret Hudson for all her hard work with Jenny's Respite and to those two loving, caring women whose Respite Care was out of this world: all our love to Lin Oldfield and her family, and to Lucy McInnes.

To all of Jenny's teachers both in elementary and high school. To Mrs. Liz Wallberg and Mr. Gee at Clarence Fulton High School in Vernon, who were both so supportive of Jenny and made her feel as though she could do all that she wanted. Mrs. Wallberg was especially persistent that Jenny publish her book. Thank you all for your belief in my daughter and for all your genuine support.

To all of Jenny's friends who accepted her for who she is, especially Lisa Rae and Cierra Carlyle and your lovely comments. As well as Sarah and Alyssa for their friendship.

Also for Kayla's friendship with Jenny.

To my family and friends who were there for me one hundred and ten percent, in all aspects of my life. Thank you for being there for me as I went through this ride with Jenny: I will always be eternally grateful. Special thank you to my sister Vicki who came to take such good care of me when I had surgery recently. You are the best.

To the wonderful people who took their time to write testimonials for my book—I am so appreciative.

To the Influence Publishing team, for believing in me and assisting me in the publication of this book. You all worked so hard, and were there for me every step of the way.

To Trista Baldwin for all her hard work on my cover design and author photo. I enjoyed all our Skype meetings and phone calls.

To Nina Shoroplova, my editor. Thank you for all your input and knowledge in editing; I have never written a book before! Thank you for helping me make this book an awesome, loving testament to Jenny.

To Temple Grandin whose story is such a huge inspiration for the autistic community, and inspiring me to encourage Jenny's ambition and talent.

To the Kaufmanns and their son Raun in Sheffield, Massachusetts, and The Son-Rise Program® team at the Autism Treatment Center of America®. Their story and programs—originally designed to support their son—have helped hundreds of parents with their autistic, special needs children. Find them www.AutismTreatment.org

Holly Robinson Pete and Jenny McCarthy; as celebrity mothers of autistic boys—thank-you for your inspiration within the autistic community, and for all that you have done through your HollyRod Foundation and as President of Generation Rescue, respectively.

Lastly and not least are my thanks to all the autistic and special needs individuals who cope with their world in society each and every day. The obstacles you have to face are amazing. Here is to your courage, hard work, and your joy for life.

Contents

Foreword

A Letter to Jenny

Jenny, we started June 1996 on a journey together, with a mother's prayer. "If only my child could tell me about her day." Jenny you were a child unable to communicate your basic needs. Anti-social, unaware of the world around you. Wow, look at you now. The changes are spectacular, Jenny. I liken you to a sponge—you seem to absorb and immerse yourself in your topic to experience and discover everything there is to know about this subject.

Jenny, you have a flair for the theatrical, like the famous actress your mother is. You have a love for music, dance, and chocolate. You are outstanding as a puppeteer.

You enjoy videos, colouring, animals, computer games, and story books.

You are determined, strong willed and compassionate with those you love. You have very strong likes and dislikes. This year you have been willing to try new foods—way to go!

You are smart, creative, adventurous, and physically strong. Playful, with a great sense of humour, and persistent; you enjoy structure, are confident, and are a leader.

Jenny, you have made incredible strides in your speech. You are truly alive in this world. Thank you for including me in your journey. It has been great and I have learned lots from you. I know you will do wonderfully in kindergarten.

Love, Gail Cunningham—Co-Owner of
Brer Rabbit Day Care (June 1998)

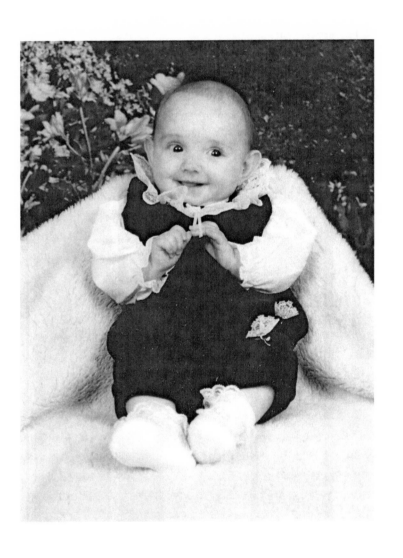

Chapter One

Jenny Story Enters the World

I remember Jenny's birth as clear as a bell. We had left Manitoba a couple of years earlier and gone off to the Land of the Northern Lights, because my then-husband had the opportunity to go to carpentry school and work in Yellowknife in the Northwest Territories.

We had been trying for five years to have a child and I thought it would be clear sailing as I had become pregnant very quickly with my son thirteen years earlier. That hadn't happened for me this time around though, as I first had a miscarriage and then found out in 1992 that I had endometriosis, which my gynecologist told me was a condition resulting from endometrial tissue outside the uterus making it hard to conceive and causing me severe abdominal and pelvic pain.

My gynecologist told me the chances of my getting pregnant with endometriosis were slim. The week before I was to fly down to Edmonton for laser surgery for the condition, I had been feeling quite nauseous and not myself, so I went to see my local doctor. When the nurse said it would be a good idea to do a pregnancy test, I actually laughed and said, "You're kidding. My gynecologist said my chances of getting pregnant are next to impossible with endometriosis."

I was so sure the test would be negative. I was sitting in the waiting room with a mixed bag of emotions. I kept saying to myself, "Stop thinking there is a glimmer of hope." But I have always been a positive person and, deep down, I was saying, "Let it be."

So there I was in the waiting room thinking about the trip to Edmonton and what I still needed to pack when the nurse walked into the waiting area with a big smile on her face and announced I was pregnant.

"What!" I exclaimed.

She told me I was four weeks along and congratulated me. Time stood still and I felt both giddy and dizzy all at once. I wondered if my ears were playing tricks on me, and if we shouldn't take another test to confirm the pregnancy. It was a surreal moment.

I was jubilant, overjoyed, crying, and then also terrified; I didn't want to go through another miscarriage. I was thirty-seven years old and my son Christopher was thirteen. I'd had such a healthy pregnancy with him that I kept positive thoughts that this third pregnancy was going to be just like his.

Every monthly checkup went well, and the baby and I were both healthy. I couldn't have asked for a better pregnancy. I did not know if the baby was a boy or a girl and I did not want to know; I wanted to be surprised but, most importantly, I wanted the baby to be healthy. Due to the way I was carrying, I was convinced I was having another boy. A lot of people thought the same. Chris would have a brother and that would be cool. Deep down though, I was thinking it would be nice if it was a girl—to have that "million dollar family" with one of each.

I was very careful about everything as I wanted to carry to term. I gained quite a bit of weight but felt really good and, wow, this baby was on the go—doing somersaults, flip flops, kicking, and moving.

I was so excited and relieved that I was making it to term.

I was out with friends late Saturday morning of February 6 when I started feeling pressure and some pain in my lower back; it grew stronger and stronger on my tailbone. I thought, "This baby is heading out the wrong way."

This was totally different from when I had been in labour with Chris. With him, I'd had really bad cramps that felt like indigestion. My due date this time was between February 6 and 8, so it was clear I was in labour. I said to everyone that we needed to grab my hospital bag from home and head off to Stanton Hospital. "This baby wants out."

We rushed to the hospital and I was checked in. What I thought was going to be a short labour turned out to be very long and intense, and I got good use out of my Lamaze® breathing techniques. I never wanted to look at ice chunks again afterwards, as I had chewed on buckets of them during those long hours.

At 1:51 a.m. on Sunday, February 7, little Jenny made her mark on this earth. She was hesitant, but finally decided it was time. When she was delivered, I said to Dr. Bhatla, "Let me hold my little boy."

He smiled and said, "Janet, she is a girl; you have a daughter."

"No, it is a boy!" I stated, and we laughed.

I was overjoyed to have a girl and declared, "Jenny, her name is Jenny Leigh." I don't know where her name came from. She was so little: 6 pounds, 5 ounces. I remember the doctor commenting on how alert she was. It was as though she was saying, "Here I am. Hello, everyone. What's happening?"

She was healthy except for a little bit of jaundice so she "sunbathed" in the incubator to assist her immature liver to do its job. She looked so adorable soaking it all in with her eye protectors on. She was a cutie pie right from the beginning. I was on top of the world and felt so blessed and grateful to have this precious daughter in my life. I couldn't wait for her to meet her big brother Chris and he couldn't wait either. When I had become pregnant with Jenny, I always made sure that Chris didn't feel left out, was included in every part of the pregnancy, and was okay with it all. The morning I gave birth to Jenny, Christopher never once left the waiting room as he wanted to be there when she was born. He stayed there all day and night—what a trooper he was. He was very excited and held her close so lovingly and cautiously, talking to her; that is a moment etched into my memory forever. I could see his love, his caring, and protectiveness right from the beginning.

I have been blessed twice with two wonderful children.

I was also blessed to have Louise Laframboise in my life—a genuine friend, neighbour, and confidante. She was there for me right from the beginning of my pregnancy; she was there with me in the labour room; and she held Jenny soon after her birth. As she had three boys, it was nice to see her with Jenny—she became her second mum when I eventually went back to work.

In the 1990s, a woman stayed in the hospital for a couple

of days after giving birth. It was really nice to get some rest after such an exhausting experience—not like nowadays when you have the baby and go home right away. After my stay in the hospital, it was good to be back in the comfort of my own home, introducing Jenny to her new life.

I tried extremely hard to breastfeed Jenny. She couldn't latch on as she had such a tiny mouth and my nipples were too big for her. I tried pumping my breast milk, but it just wasn't working. She was losing weight, and when the public health nurse and my doctor recommended that I switch to formula, I did exactly that. It was the best decision for Jenny as well as for me, as I was losing energy and sleep. Once she started adjusting and liking the formula milk from the bottle, things became normal. I remember the night feeds vividly—it was just me and her, bonding together; me feeding her and then rocking her off to sleep in the rocking chair. Those were beautiful moments, being with her; more memories etched in my mind.

As time went on, Jenny blossomed. She was tiny but full of spunk. As the doctor had commented, she was very alert and lively. She crawled and walked very early, always exploring and wanting to see what everything was and how it worked. I remember walking in on Jenny and Chris once when he was sending her like a sling shot in the Jolly Jumper®—she was loving every second of it and had the hugest smile on her face, laughing so hard. So was her brother Chris, until he saw me with my eyes and mouth wide open in horror and the veins sticking out on my neck. Even though she loved it, I made sure that didn't happen again. She had no fear, that is for sure.

Jenny adored playing with Chris and vice versa. He was so good with her—they love each other so much and have a wonderful bond. He has been the sweetest, kindest, most protective brother a sister could have. If ever I forgot something when I was bathing her or needed help, Chris was always there. I have a picture of the two of them after a bath, with our dog Dino next to them; Chris always ensured Dino behaved so that Jenny was safe. He liked to play with her and her toys, and read her favourite stories. He was a very selfless boy, and understood I needed to spend a great deal of time taking care of his baby sister.

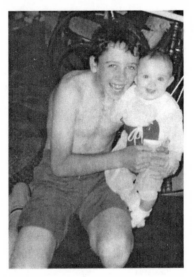

Chris and Jenny love the Jolly Jumper®.

Jenny was always investigating something, always on a mission. She loved to get in my cupboards and play with the spoons, and the pots and pans. She was quite the social butterfly too. She would go to anyone, and loved playing with other children.

Jenny's health and development was all it should be and I was over the moon with happiness at seeing her flourish.

Chapter Two

Where Did Jenny Go?

In wanting to be a good mother and do the utmost and best for my child I made sure Jenny had a good diet, slept well, got lots of fresh air, and had opportunities to make friends. I was there for her one hundred percent in every avenue of her life. She was not a sickly child. She had the odd cold and earache; however, nothing really bad.

I knew that childhood vaccines are very important. I'd had my son's all done and naturally would follow suit with Jenny. I never thought anything of it; I was being a responsible mum. I loved my daughter and was doing the best for her health. It was difficult to see my child react each time the needle was given, but Jenny was my little trooper.

It was time for Jenny's twelve-month shot, so off we went to the clinic. Chris, Jenny, and I went out of town that day, but later that night on our way home, I knew there was something wrong with her. She was getting too warm and becoming ill. By the time we got home she was worse, vomiting with diarrhea. Everything was coming out of both ends and she was losing energy. As my then-husband was out of town, I dropped Chris off at my friend Louise's house and took Jenny to the hospital.

Being February in Yellowknife, it was extremely cold. I really had to bundle her up—between her being so feverish and then heading out into the harsh weather, I was worried. When I got to the hospital, I felt a sense of relief that a doctor would see her and let me know what was going on. The doctor was an intern. He looked at me and said matter-of-factly, "Yes, she has a fever; she has probably caught some bug. Give her some Pedialyte®," and he sent me back home.

When we returned home, however, I was still unsettled because she was not getting better; she became worse and was like a rag doll. She was still vomiting—couldn't keep anything down—the diarrhea was like water and she was burning up. I said, "To heck with this!"

I went back to the hospital and refused to leave. This time, another doctor said to the nurses, "Get her right away into a room," and he started doing tests.

It was hell for me to wait alone outside the room, having my little one rushed away and not knowing what was going on—I was beside myself and in tears. I knew I had to be strong, however. I had to buck up, even though deep down I was frantic and my heart was leaping out of my chest. I was praying to God not to let her go.

I kept repeating over and over, "She is so special; it took me so long to have her; please let her be okay."

One of the tests they did was for spinal meningitis. I found out later that when they examined her spinal fluid, they found her white blood cells were completely out of whack. My motherly intuition was right. I knew it was really serious and not just a common fever with sickness. Soon she was on an IV, with more tests being done.

Jenny was in the hospital for over a week. I spent close to twenty-four hours a day there, sleeping right beside her. I never left the room for long, except to spend time with Chris, as this was as hard on him as it was on me. With my then-husband being away for schooling, Chris stayed with Louise and her family, which I appreciated so much; they were a godsend. I would check on him often, as he needed my love and attention too. I knew Chris was really worried, as was Louise.

During the week Jenny was in the hospital, the doctor could not tell me definitely what the problem had been. A virus? They weren't sure. It was a mystery. It daunted me that they couldn't say specifically what had made her so sick. However, she gradually regained her health and energy; her appetite grew and the fever lessened. She was physically getting back to herself and that is what mattered. I could breathe a sigh of relief. The doctor gave us the go-ahead to go back home. What a great feeling.

Even so, never getting a firm diagnosis on what had caused her to be so sick didn't sit well with me. Our family wasn't sick and we hadn't been around anyone who was. No illnesses were going around the community that were a cause for concern and, with the freezing temperatures, bugs and viruses died right away.

Regardless, the comfort and joy of being back home again took over. Being in our own environment, getting back to our normal lives and enjoying each day knowing Jenny was with us gave us peace of mind. I know for Chris as well it felt so good to be together again. Jenny went back to Louise for daycare, while I went back to work.

We were looking forward to enjoying happy days ahead, or so we thought.

As time went on, Jenny was very good physically. However, her mental wellbeing and socializing were visibly different from before she was ill. At first, I didn't say anything to anyone, as I thought I must be overreacting. After a while though, I knew something was seriously wrong. She had stopped making eye contact with me; she would not say the few words she had learned; she was not sociable anymore ... she seemed to be in a world of her own. Chris had noticed the change as well, and was puzzled and worried about it. He told me, "She's not saying her words or looking at me—she doesn't play like she used to."

I thought maybe something was wrong with Jenny's hearing. I took her for testing, but she got very upset and had a tantrum; she could not handle the situation. I wondered whether she was going through a phase as this was so out of character for her. But each day it was the same scenario with no improvement and I couldn't understand what was happening. My head was spinning as we had already gone through the horror of her being sick and almost losing her, and I kept praying that she was not experiencing something new. I kept telling myself, "It's just a phase. It will pass, and she will be back to her usual self."

So I went on with my daily life, working as a dental hygienist at the Yellowknife Dental Clinic.

One day, when I walked into Louise's house to pick up Jenny, I was struck by the distraught look on Louise's face. My heart dropped as I thought, "My God, something has happened to Jenny. Is she hurt or suddenly ill?"

Louise asked me to come into the kitchen with her. From a distance, I could see Jenny had many figurines lined up in a specific order, which she had been doing frequently at home. Louise looked at me with concern and said, "I do not know who that is in there, but it is not Jenny. Where did Jenny go?"

To hear my friend say this was actually a huge relief, followed by fear. I confided in Louise that I knew something was not right, that Jenny was different from before. I told my friend that the change had been driving me crazy. I now had to face this and get her checked to see what was happening to my little girl.

Just as I was planning to take Jenny to the doctor and have her checked out, I received a phone call from my mother Vera. I remember screaming and falling to the floor. My father had suddenly passed away. I was devastated and heartbroken, as my dad was a very special man in my life. I had always enjoyed our talks and outings. I thank God that he had met Jenny only a few months earlier. I look at the pictures now with him holding Jenny on his knee and they make me cry with happiness. Dad was like a second father to my son, as I had been a single parent for a while with Chris; Dad and Mum were always there for him.

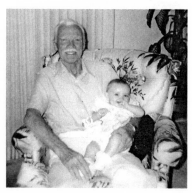

At my parents' home in White Rock, Jenny sits on Grandpa Bob's lap.

We drove the 2,330 kilometres from Yellowknife to White Rock, British Columbia. I felt numb before, during, and after Dad's funeral. It didn't sink in that he was actually gone. I treasure the memory of our times together so dearly.

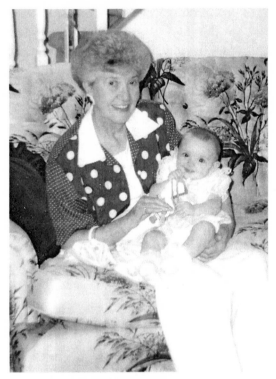

Jenny sits on Nana Vera's lap.

We'd been in Yellowknife for four years when my then-husband and I decided to move to Vernon to be closer to my mum in White Rock. White Rock was too expensive for us and Vernon was only five hours away. It had a good feel and was very family oriented—a good area to be raising Chris and Jenny. I was very drawn to the Okanagan

Valley: the landscape, the lakes, and the beauty. The main attraction, however, was their larger medical centre where I hoped to learn more about the sudden change in Jenny.

When I look back now, I realize it was the best decision I ever made, especially for Jenny—Vernon was our "saviour city." It was a hard decision on Chris though, as he was fourteen, an exceptionally difficult age to move away from friends and the life he knew in Yellowknife. As a teenager he was heading to a strange city, meeting new peers, and facing new challenges.

We sold our home in Yellowknife and on October 6, 1994 we drove to Vernon. We did not have a place yet, so we stayed in a motel until we found a house a couple of weeks later. We picked an area near the huge park and kids playground at Kin Beach on Okanagan Lake, which was essentially our front yard. We became a permanent fixture on the beach year-round, as Jenny took to the water like a dolphin—she was becoming such a strong swimmer. We spent hours in the lake knocking each other off the floats and throwing the frisbee back and forth. We loved Vernon's waterfront and lakes, and spent a great deal of time at Paddlewheel Park and Kal Beach. At Paddlewheel, we'd always swim out to the diving platform in the middle of the lake and jump off it over and over again. I also took her to the water slides a lot—she adored the tube slides and the pool. She loved all the equipment and swings at the playground too, but had absolutely no fear of heights, which was terrifying for me—I needed to be exceptionally attentive and by her side at all times.

Jenny's unexplained behaviour continued to worsen during this time. She wouldn't talk at all anymore, preferring to just grunt with her head down. She still lined objects up meticulously and, Heaven forbid if anyone should interfere with the order. She would spin herself in circles constantly and refuse to stop. She would only eat certain foods, which would last for months until I could introduce something else. Her five senses—to light, sound, touch, taste, and smell—were highly sensitive ... much more than the average.

Additionally, she had begun having fits if we didn't take the exact same route on our walks through the park, or if we didn't step on the exact same stones. She even became upset when we altered our driving route—any change of routine was met with extreme resistance. The fits were so severe that I took to giving her frequent baths, as being in water appeared to calm her down. She had grown very strong so the fits were sucking my energy dry as they occurred more than once a day. I was devastated when she started hitting and biting herself, and throwing herself around.

I felt so bad for her. It was extremely emotional for me to watch my child experience such despair, and I tried hard to stay calm and be present for her so she would be comforted enough to stop. She would have fits in stores if we didn't go down the same aisle as we had previously; the fits garnered reactions of disgust from other shoppers. Some people would even say to me, "What a bad girl. She needs a spanking, the spoiled brat."

One day while walking through the playground, we deviated from our normal route, and Jenny launched into a full-on blow-up. I couldn't contain her when I tried to pick her up, as she was thrashing around so violently, hitting and biting, all the while hollering loudly. I was already exhausted from an earlier episode that morning and it took everything in me to try to get her to the edge of the park. All the people around us stopped and stared. But I didn't care what they thought—I just wanted to shield my little girl from herself, get her home and into the bath, to try to calm her down.

It was at that point that Chris's friend Justin Dorval came running up to me, having observed us struggling. He said, "It's okay, Janet. I will take her."

Justin is a strong guy; however, he was very delicate with her and held her comfortably so she would not hurt herself, and kept her as calm as possible. All the while he was making sure I was okay and could make it home. I was taking deep breaths and trying to collect myself. Thank God he came by when he did. To this day, I still thank Justin for his help that afternoon.

Jenny's fits were very hard on Chris as well. It was alarming for him whenever she started hurting herself, and he always tried to help me calm her down by holding her for me, or helping to put her in the bath. He felt helpless at times but so wanted to be there for her (which he always was and is) and he would do his best to soothe her. He would put on a movie, play songs she liked, or play with her on the floor with her favourite toys and stuffed animals. He felt so sorry for what she was going through and wanted her back as she was before.

Chris really didn't like the way people reacted or made comments about Jenny when she became upset about a scenario and had a fit in public. He knew she was a sweetheart and not the "bad girl" strangers would assume she was. One night I took them both out for supper. It had been a while and we wanted to try again, as Jenny needed to adjust to being out in public. Unfortunately, Jenny was not at all comfortable in the restaurant—Chris and I thought maybe it was the lights, the volume of the noise, the unfamiliar surroundings and people. We were trying to settle her down with her favourite stuffed toy and colouring books, but she just grabbed everything and climbed under the table. People were giving us odd looks, and we did our best to coax Jenny out so she would join us and eat her food, but she was becoming increasingly upset. Chris finally looked at me and said, "It's okay, Mum, you eat."

He joined Jenny under the table and made her feel comfy by calmly talking to her and playing with her for a bit. Slowly, he got her to come out and sit with us, holding her as she started to eat alongside him. I looked at him and thought how fortunate I am to have such a wonderful son; how lucky Jenny is to have a brother like Chris. I was moved to tears, and the picture of the two of them together that day will forever be etched in my mind. He didn't care what other people thought and how they were staring at us, he only wanted to make sure his little sister and his mom were okay. He reassured me that those people were just cruel and ignorant.

Jenny's fits were horrible. My heart ached for her, as she couldn't help them. I realize kids will be kids, but Jenny's behaviour was abnormal to the extreme. This was not her former personality at all—she was not the girl she had been before the illness.

Chapter Three

My Dream Team

Thankfully, I managed to get in to see a doctor in Vernon relatively quickly. I will not mention his name, as over the period of time we saw him, he was not medically there for my daughter and me. When I explained to this doctor the history and concerns I had about Jenny's behaviour since she'd been sick—that she was not her normal self—he looked at me as though I was simply an overly reactive, overboard mother.

The doctor told me Jenny was just slow to develop. "She will talk eventually. Kids are kids." His reactions and facial expressions said, "Let's just get this mum out of here."

He suggested taking her for a hearing test. I explained we'd tried to do that in Yellowknife but she was uncooperative; however, I would definitely try again if it was going to help me figure out what was going on. It wasn't much, but it was a start. I was really upset on the way home because of how the doctor had treated me. He was very rude, and made me feel like an overly neurotic mother.

I took Jenny to the Public Health Unit for a hearing test. They tried, along with my help, to get a test, but the fits were on and Jenny wouldn't stay still, nor would she listen—she just flapped her hands, screamed, and tried to run out of the room. She also couldn't talk, so she couldn't understand or even gesture to tell us if she could hear or not. She exhausted both the audiologist and me. There was no way we could do a proper test on her hearing to reveal anything.

I looked down at my little sweetie as we walked away from the clinic, her face all red and sweating, and I felt so sorry for her. I needed to get to the root of the problem for her sake, as she needed and deserved appropriate care. She hadn't asked for this to happen to her; it was not her fault.

I have never been known as an "assertive person," but I demanded that this doctor refer Jenny to a pediatrician, as her behaviour was definitely not normal. He was none too impressed, but I wanted to make sure she got the best care. That's how we started with Dr. Eiko Waida, a pediatrician in Vernon about whom I had heard very encouraging things. I was looking forward to meeting her and seeing if she could shed light on what was happening with Jenny. I was looking for an answer, a ray of sunshine, an opening for Jenny and me to peek through.

We met with Dr. Waida, and explained to her how none of Jenny's strange behaviour was apparent before becoming ill after the vaccination. I described the fits of rage when her routine was altered, how she would grunt and push me when she wanted things, how she would line up toys in specific ways and allow no one to alter or touch or play with them. I explained how she would only watch certain movies, over and over again: *Fox and the Hound* and *Thumbelina*. She knew them off by heart (and consequently, so did I).

I relayed that she was very sensitive to lights and loud noises and did not like people hugging, touching, being close to her, or being in her personal space. If she did not like something she would act up and get very upset. She was untrusting. She was always lost in her own world and I was left wondering where she was and what was going on in her mind.

I told Dr. Waida how worried I was when Jenny would harm herself if anything was altered, if we deviated from routine, or if one of her five senses bothered her. I explained that baths would calm Jenny down but that I had to do this several times a day, and looking after her had become a twenty-four-hour job, which took every ounce of my energy. This level of care was exhausting for me and I knew I needed to be healthy and alert for her, but I accepted the fatigue as I wanted to support her one hundred and ten percent. I admitted her care was taking its toll, because I was on my own (now separated from my then-husband) with my son and daughter to take care of in addition to working a full-time job.

Dr. Waida listened attentively, and observed Jenny closely. She tested her social behaviour, her speech, and her ability to converse and interact with others. She tested how she played with toys and behaved with books. She asked how Jenny was with visual learning. When Dr. Waida started to do some tests, Jenny became agitated and had one of her fits. After an hour, Dr. Waida took my hand. She actually hugged me and said, "This girl needs to be assessed right away. With the behaviour I am seeing, I am leaning toward a diagnosis of Autism and Pervasive Development Delay.

And then you, my dear, need respite."

Autism. Pervasive Development Delay. I did not know what these terms meant. Dr. Waida assured me that things would become clearer in time, and that she would put me in contact with the appropriate organizations and care services—anything and anyone who could help Jenny.

I asked her what she meant when she referenced Respite. She explained, "Janet, it is some time and space given to you to be by yourself, so you can fuel yourself up and get reenergized both physically and mentally."

I responded, "Oh, that is not necessary. I am her mum and should always be the one by her side, as I know her better than anyone else."

However, deep down, I knew she was right; I badly needed the respite.

Dr. Waida informed me that Jenny would be placed on a waiting list to be assessed by specialists in Vancouver, but I knew we had to get something going for her right away. I wanted to do everything I could to help Jenny as soon as possible.

The Dream Team

I call this circle of people our "Dream Team," as each of them became instrumental in Jenny's development. They did everything possible to help her grow and thrive, going the extra mile (or ten!) to do everything the specialists recommended. We have become so close; they are like our second family.

Darlene Wolsey

Our Dream Team began forming in June 1996 when I met the lovely, caring Darlene Wolsey from the Community Child Care Options Program. She is a gem of a woman.

When Darlene first met Jenny, she could not interact with her socially. Jenny was in her own world, grunting for things, and making no eye contact. Darlene observed Jenny moving repetitively and spinning herself in circles, becoming agitated when we tried to stop her—to save her from falling down—having fits if her toys were not in the lineup she wanted.

After we discussed what I was up against with Jenny, Darlene quickly identified that there were ongoing difficulties with transitions, especially to new environments and new people. Jenny was very wary of strangers and it took quite some time to win her trust. Darlene found that Jenny responded best and felt safest when she was given the opportunity to move through transitions with support from someone she felt comfortable with. That person needed to understand her language abilities and give her time to adjust to the change. When Jenny wasn't provided with this, she would feel overwhelmed and very anxious. She would withdraw, have fits, and be uncooperative and tearful.

Darlene felt that it would be most fruitful and advantageous for Jenny to go into a normal daycare. It was something she had been wanting to try out with a special needs child and see if it could be successful. She suggested we look at Brer Rabbit Day Care.

Gail Cunningham, Deb Radies, Shelley Burrill, and the Staff of
Brer Rabbit Day Care

The next people who joined our Dream Team were truly a godsend—absolute blessings for Jenny and me. These angels are Gail Cunningham and Deb Radies, who operated the wonderful Brer Rabbit Day Care. I cannot say enough about Gail and Deb. They are the most caring, loving, genuine, and hard-working women I have ever met. Their daycare was one in a million and I always thank God for bringing them into Jenny's and my lives. They were so welcoming to my little girl, so patient and giving. I felt their sincerity in my gut the instant I met them.

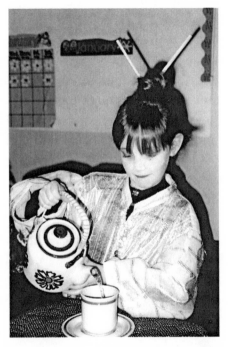

Jenny dresses in a kimono for Japanese Day at
Brer Rabbit Day Care.

Brer Rabbit Day Care was an open, well-organized facility with warm inviting colours on the walls, and I felt instantly at home. Everyone had their own locker area and there were pictures of the children decorating the walls. It had great playground equipment in a huge yard, including a big treehouse. There were pools for the kids in warm weather and a covered outdoor area for them to eat and do crafts. They made crafts tenfold—such lovely inventive things. They often had visitors come to talk and teach the children. There were endless educational outings and fun adventures to many different places, ensuring the children learned during their time there.

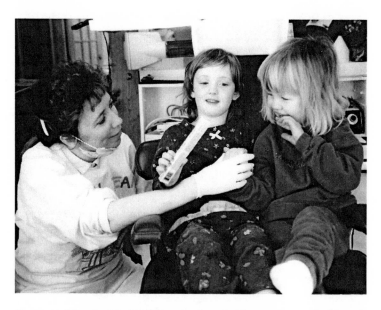

Jenny and her buddy Maddie on a Brer Rabbit outing to the dental clinic where I worked.

I so appreciated the fabulous variety of educational toys at the daycare and they were always bringing in new ones to maintain the children's interest. They had movie time, snack time, nap time, and so much more—I was truly in awe. I wish I could have gone there myself as a child.

Above everything I loved about Brer Rabbit, I appreciated Gail's and Deb's engagement with Jenny. They were genuinely invested in her wellbeing and wanted to know everything about her—how to make sure she felt comfortable so she could trust them, and how to ensure her environment would be mentally and physically safe. They were there for her every step of the way. I explained how important routine was to her, and that she grunted for help instead of asking, and played in her own world. I described the circumstances that often resulted in fits and explained that she didn't want to socialize, always seeming far away in thought.

In the beginning, Gail, Deb, and their staff had their hands full taking care of Jenny. The first day was excruciating for me as she was crying and screaming, and I thought, "What am I doing? I cannot do this. I am a terrible mother, leaving her when she has special needs because of her autism."

However, in talking with Gail and the other caregivers, a reassuring feeling came over me and I knew these women would be genuinely loving and caring with Jenny. Gail gave me a hug and said, "Everything will be fine; you'll see."

I vividly remember saying to Gail that day how much I would love it if Jenny could say, "Hi, Mum. How are you?" or tell me about her day when I came to pick her up. Gail and I still reminisce about that wish to this day.

The Brer Rabbit Day Care staff had to deal with the fits

Jenny had in many different scenarios—in play situations, with loud sounds, having a lot of people around, and eating the meals they prepared (Jenny was such a picky eater and her sense of taste was so heightened). Being with kids at a daycare was hard for her; their noise and playfulness would throw her off and make her upset. As she did not talk, she would get frustrated when she couldn't communicate, and have a fit. Everyone at Brer Rabbit was extremely patient with Jenny. They worked around her needs, always communicating with her, and ensuring she was safe and not hurting herself.

It was a total blessing when Brer Rabbit hired Shelley Burrill to become—as I called her—"Jenny's second Mum." Shelley was with Jenny constantly, offering her a sense of security and helping her understand her environment, while assisting her in socializing and communicating with other children and workers. Shelley gently guided her in coming out of her inner world, and watching what her peers were doing around her. She slowly encouraged Jenny to play and interact with the other children, despite Jenny's desire to play by herself in her own world, where she felt happy and comfortable. Jenny would become very upset, tearful, and quite loud if children tried to take toys from her line up, or remove something she wanted to play with. She needed extensive support in new environments, to learn new routines, and meet expectations required of her.

Darlene from Community Child Care Options worked with me, Shelley, and the women at Brer Rabbit to establish individual programs to accommodate Jenny's needs. Jenny's difficulties in receptive and expressive language made it challenging for her to understand and follow directions and routines, and to decipher social rules. Shelley tirelessly went the extra mile with Jenny, enabling me to go to work each day knowing that she was looking out for Jenny in every way possible.

Over the course of her first year at Brer, Jenny would constantly watch, copy, and imitate the other children's actions—both physically and in speech—regardless of whether the behaviour she witnessed was positive or negative. Shelley told me when Jenny's friend Maddie went into the pool off a dangerous edge and was given "alone time," Jenny became upset and proceeded to do exactly what Maddie had done. Shelley also pointed out how loving Jenny could be—when she and Jenny bumped heads, Jenny would put Shelley's head in her hands and ask "Are you okay?"

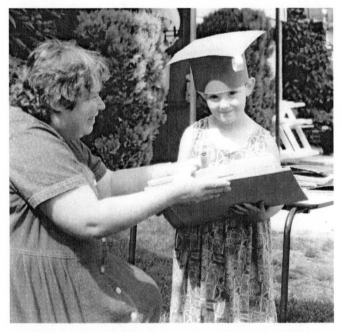

Jenny receives her diploma and scrapbook from Gail at the Brer Rabbit Day Care Graduation Day Ceremony, June 1997.

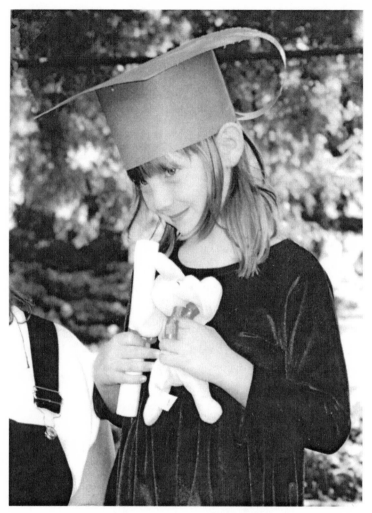

Jenny graduates from Brer Rabbit Day Care.

Two big memories come to mind about Gail and Deb and their daycare. First is the annual graduation day they had for the children and their parents every June. The work and preparation the Brer Rabbit staff did—like the decorations, the actual ceremony, and the food they laid out for everyone—were truly amazing and took my breath away. The children wore graduation hats and each child would go up separately for Gail to say something about the child and their year and then give them a diploma. It was so sweet. This is one of the examples of their genuine love for the children in their care.

The other memory is the scrapbooks they did every year for each child. These books held scores of pictures to take us parents through a visual journey of what they had done all year, both inside and outside daycare. The books also held all their craft work, the pictures they had drawn, certificates, and so much more. It was truly like being with them every day and sharing the moments. I could see the growth in Jenny from year to year. I can never thank them enough for these scrapbooks, as it is hard for a parent to be away from her child, but sometimes circumstances don't allow anything else. I cherish those physical memories.

Jenny and I have taken them out through the years and we sit down and look at them. They make us laugh and cry with the memories that come flooding back. This would have taken a lot of time to do and they did it with so much love. Gail and Deb are two wonderful and gracious women.

Fran Wood

Darlene from Community Child Care Options also introduced us to one of the first professionals to join our Dream Team. Fran Wood was a Play Therapist who worked out of the Public Health Unit in Vernon.

Our first meeting was memorable. I came out of it completely drained, as did Fran. Fran started by suggesting we try having Jenny join her in the playroom area (unaccompanied by me) while I watched from another room through a one-way mirror. It was an experience I will never forget.

Fran began by trying to get Jenny to talk and play with her. Jenny, however, moved as far away from Fran as she could, and became fixated on one toy. Then Jenny had her first fit with screaming, yelling, kicking, throwing herself, and hitting herself and Fran. Jenny reacted very negatively to every attempt Fran made, grunting loudly, pushing Fran away, throwing things, and avoiding all verbal and eye contact.

I watched in horror as my heart cried out not only for Jenny but for Fran as well. She was a lovely woman who was doing her best to connect with Jenny. The tantrums got worse as Jenny could not handle any of it. They were both sweating profusely and had faces the colour of bright red tomatoes, while I bawled on the other side of the mirror. Eventually Fran stopped trying, as Jenny was not trusting nor wanting to be in there.

When I went back into the room, Fran said, "I do not know how you have been able to handle this day in and day out."

Fran explained that she would have regular play therapy—Theraplay®—sessions with Jenny, and that she would go to Jenny's daycare so Jenny would be in an environment she knew, making their time together more comfortable for her. Gail and Deb agreed, and observing Fran helped them in working with Jenny as well. Through Fran, Jenny was encouraged to move toward healthy play and to socialize properly with the other children. A lot of time, patience, and a variety of techniques were required for everyone to accomplish this—from the daycare staff, Fran, me, and (primarily) Jenny—but play therapy was eventually a successful approach.

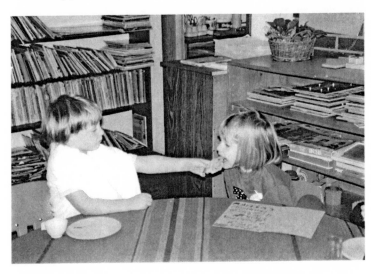

Jenny (on the left) takes part in Theraplay at Brer Rabbit Day Care.

After almost a year of working together, Fran reported that Jenny still had very significant development delays, and she suspected Jenny had autism because of her "Pervasive Development Delay." Fran said that Jenny was making tremendous progress, but that this progress was fragile, and Jenny would continue to require support services. She found Jenny's greatest difficulties were in the areas of language and social skills. She explained that it was often difficult to ascertain what would start Jenny's tantrums and how difficult she could be to settle. She said Jenny was not an easy child to parent in that she was not always "readable" and "responsive." She felt Jenny needed to be with adults who could care for her, providing consistency, routine, structure, and a calm approach.

In conclusion, she stated that Jenny was a complex child and that I was doing everything I could and had successfully put a team in place in which all members were working collaboratively. She also stressed that it was very important all caregivers knew how to deal with Jenny's behaviour and how to communicate with her to ensure continued development. Jenny slowly started to settle into the play therapy with Fran, which offered me greater insight into how to help her with communication and how to handle her fits. I appreciated learning the Theraplay® techniques from Fran, as I could incorporate them at home.

Lisa Coley-Donahue

Next on my Dream Team list is Lisa Coley-Donahue, a Speech and Language Pathologist, and an amazing woman. Like the rest of the team, she is very giving, very caring, and was there for Jenny in every way she could be. She also went to Brer Rabbit to work with Jenny, understanding the benefits of a familiar environment. Again, this also helped Gail, Deb, and Shelley learn ways to improve Jenny's speech and language development.

Lisa was aware that Jenny was suspected of being autistic. She saw that Jenny was very dependent on me and her special needs workers at the daycare, particularly Shelley who assisted in conveying Jenny's wants and desires. At this point, Jenny was verbalizing in an imitative fashion, known as echolalia. Lisa saw this and explained that Jenny's echolalia was highly automatic and frequently non-functional.

Lisa pointed out that Jenny's understanding of language was severely limited, as she was unable to respond spontaneously, explain, make requests, or participate in conversations. I am incredibly grateful to Lisa for establishing a process to help Jenny communicate and understand the simplest words, items, and objects, which enabled her to begin interacting and sharing with her peers. As I was with Jenny for all Lisa's appointments, I learned a great deal about language.

Initially, Jenny responded as usual in a different surrounding with a different person. I commend Lisa, as it took special patience, care, and specific avenues for her to use her professional skills and lovely personality to not upset Jenny and have her launch into one of her fits. Jenny required routine and consistency from her caregivers, and most importantly a calm temperament in dealing with her behaviour. This is key for a child and their parent—it makes the whole journey more comfortable, and offers a light at the end of a dark tunnel; a rainbow ending in a pot of gold for the child and her future. I use these comparisons frequently when relaying our adventure to other people, as they capture how I've felt through it all. Jenny is an example of this journey.

We grew very close to Lisa. It was hard initially to watch Jenny experience her temper tantrums as they involved throwing herself to the floor, banging her head, screaming, and crying. Lisa said it was difficult to predict antecedent events to these behaviours. Sometimes, there was really no clue as to what set her off. We did figure out that she reacted very strongly if one of her five senses was overstimulated. She also did not like to be hugged or touched, and needed to trust a person before she would look at them or interact with them.

Dr. Bruce Pipher

Next on the Dream Team is Dr. Bruce Pipher, Jenny's Child and Adolescent Psychiatrist, a key player in diagnosing Jenny and in providing guidance and support for Jenny and me. Our initial meeting with him was a consultation on July 3, 1998 in his Kelowna office, fifty-three kilometres south of Vernon. He agreed with the diagnosis of Mild Mentally Challenged, but he also found she had a neuropsychiatric condition that affected her social, emotional, communicative, and cognitive development. Essentially, autism. He found she had severe behavioural challenges that required extensive resources including speech and play therapy.

He tried to start a conversation with her about school and what subjects she liked, and about family and friends. She was her usual hesitant self, so he didn't push it on this first meeting with Jenny. While he was talking to me and getting information, Jenny was colouring, drawing, and playing with toys. Dr. Pipher would observe her from time to time while we talked. But he also tried to get Jenny to talk with him so he could assess her mental, social, and language skills. He then provided a report that would offer insight to Jenny's other support workers and to me, enabling us to tailor our approaches when assisting her developmentally.

Dr. Pipher was a genuine and caring doctor who went the extra mile for Jenny at every appointment she had with him. He gave her plenty of time and made sure never to rush her, so that she was comfortable. He identified every aspect of what was going on for her so she could get the continued support she needed. Patient and kind, he was always checking in with me to ensure I was okay, and he included me in the assessment process, valuing my observations and input. He was professional and personable all in one.

Son-Rise Program®

Last, and certainly not least, is the place and the people I researched outside Canada—The Son-Rise Program® in Sheffield, Massachusetts. I discovered them when I found out and finally understood what Jenny was experiencing. I did some research on my own and one night I watched a movie called *Son-Rise: A Miracle of Love*. It was a true story made into a movie about the life of Raun Kaufman and his parents Barry Neil and Samahria Kaufman. They were told in the early 1970s that their son was severely and incurably autistic, and even though they were advised to institutionalize him because of his "hopeless, lifelong condition," the Kaufmans instead designed an innovative home-based, child-centred program in an attempt to reach their little boy. Their unique program transformed Raun from a mute, withdrawn child to a highly verbal and socially active boy with a near genius IQ. While bearing no traces of his former condition, Raun graduated from an Ivy League University and went on to become a director at an educational centre for school age children. A big difference from what would have happened if he had been placed in institutional care.

A key recommendation from The Son-Rise Program® is to join in with your child's repetitive and ritualistic behaviour, as I remember they did with Raun. They said it was the very key to unlocking the mysteries of those behaviours, and it facilitated eye contact, social development, and the inclusion of others in play. After I read this, I started joining in with Jenny all the time at home and, though it did not happen overnight, eventually Jenny's eyes began to observe what I was doing, and even at times met my gaze. To see that beautiful smile of hers appear, and to look directly into her beautiful big blue eyes was the most incredible feeling I could have had. This was also passed on to the caregivers and professionals working with her.

I always have said that Jenny is "Normal with Special Needs" and that other children are "Normal with no Special Needs." It's so important for us to believe in our children, to be their rock, and to go the extra mile for them; See that light at the end of the dark tunnel, catch that rainbow and all its colours; Grab that pot of gold for the future life, goals, and dreams of our children.

I have included more about how and why the Kaufmans' story resonated with me in Appendix A. Their story is truly inspiring, and offers incredible insight for caregivers of autistic children.

Chapter Four

Family Support

Chris

Chris is Jenny's older brother, born on November 9, 1979, so there are thirteen years between him and Jenny. He is now thirty-five and has grown into an amazing man and individual. I am very proud of him and happy for the life he has made for himself, which for the last nine years has been in Australia with his lovely wife Ally. And even though Chris lives so far away he Skypes regularly and he and Jenny have many conversations talking about each other's lives and other topics. They are both avid gamers so that is a huge common ground for them. Chris is also awesome at drawing and had actually started to write a book when he was in high school, which I would love him to get back to.

Growing up, Chris had no problem looking after Jenny if I needed to go out, and I always knew she was in good hands. He would pick her up from daycare for me or take her to Respite Care when needed. He loves his sister, and always enjoyed teasing her and going into her room to bug her by not leaving. They'd wrestle and he'd tease her about boys, which really ruffled her feathers. They would watch TV and movies together, and play board games. No one could ever be mean to Jenny or make her feel bad when he was around. He is very protective of Jenny, and whenever something happened in her life, he wanted to know about it.

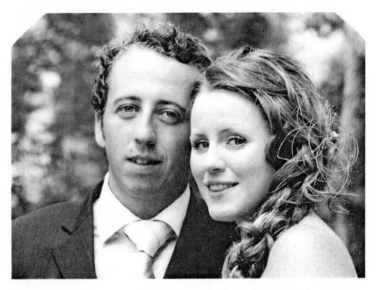

Chris and his wife Ally smile on their wedding day in Australia.

Chris has always said that if anything ever happened to me he would leave Australia in a heartbeat and come back to live in Canada to be there for Jenny. His love for his sister is undeniable and from day one has always been genuine, sincere and loving. This is the type of human being he was, as a boy, a teenager, and as the young man he has grown up to be. A role model as a son, brother, husband, and person.

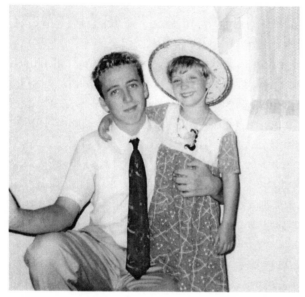

Chris and Jenny head out on a family outing.

Travis

There was a change in our family environment when Jenny was four years old. I was a single mum in the middle of a divorce, as I had been separated from my husband for two years. I had no intention of meeting anyone new at the time, but in September 1997 I met Travis, and we instantly clicked. He got along with Chris right away, and the bond he and Jenny formed was amazing.

When Travis first met Jenny he really liked her, and though it took her so long to begin trusting anyone, she was drawn to him immediately. I remember Travis telling me that Jenny looked him in the eyes and made a smile like she was saying, "I like you." He felt privileged that he was allowed into her world. I was delighted when she jumped on the coach beside him and started babbling to him incoherently—he just talked back to her normally and they proceeded to have quite the chat.

We would go to the mall and he would take her to the toy area and play with her, showing her how some of the toys worked. He was very patient and kind to her. Over time they grew closer, as Travis showed her endless love, care, kindness, and loyalty. He made a point to understand her autism and special needs, and avoided hugging her or doing anything he knew might upset her until she was ready for it. He was always there for her regardless of the challenges, and stuck by her when anyone was mean or hurt her feelings. Travis had known there was something going on with Jenny but never once backed away or said he couldn't handle it. He was there every step of the way and loved her as if she were his own, and Jenny grew to refer to him as her dad.

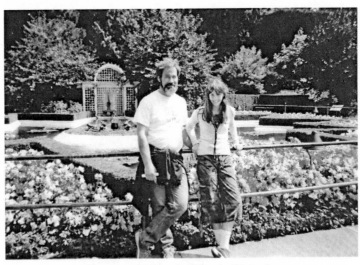

Travis and Jenny holiday in Victoria.

Travis would give me breaks by reading bedtime stories to her at night, taking her to daycare (and later school), and they had some cool games they would play together. One of her favourites was when they played "riding the bull," where Jenny would get on his shoulders and he would pretend he was bucking her off, which would cause peals of laughter on her part. He left the disciplining to me, however, when she had fits. He respected I was the mum and knew best how to respond.

Jenny was very protective of Travis. When she was four years old, he was working under his truck and she wanted to be outside with him. He told her she could not be right under the truck with him, but, she could sit close by. So she sat by the end of his legs and put her hand on his legs. A friend came by to help Travis and Jenny piped up, "No" to him; she did not want him talking or bugging her dad. Travis, his friend, and I had quite a chuckle about this. I could see as Jenny got older it became harder for Travis as she will always be his little girl and Jenny would tell him not to be calling her "Little Bear" and "Munchkin" when they were out in public, although she allowed it at home as she knew it meant a lot to him. He remains a very proud and supportive father.

Mr. Sparkles

The final member of our family support is the silent hero, Jenny's dog Mr. Sparkles. A loyal best friend and faithful companion, he has truly helped Jenny through her uphill climb in life with his big loving licks, always waiting for her when she came home, and jumping on her to play with him. He has been by her side from the moment she met him.

We had gone to view some Jack Russell puppies that were in a large pen. The parents were both short-haired Jack Russells and we thought all the puppies looked like their parents, until we saw some movement in the corner. Hiding in the back was a long-haired puppy with black colouring in addition to the beige and white sported by the rest of the litter. Jenny and I watched as this little puppy started to slowly and carefully make his way toward us, clambering over the pile of other puppies who were jumping up and down rambunctiously. He headed straight for Jenny and snuggled himself under her arm and stayed there. Jenny fell in love with him instantly, and when the owner told us he was the runt Jenny did not understand and said, "He is not called Runt, his name is Sparkles." That was the moment Sparkles joined our family.

Whenever Jenny had a bad day or issues, Sparkles would sense it and go right to her side. He was always there to cheer her up, calm her tears, and make her smile. His love and licks put her in a whole different frame of mind and made her forget her woes. He was a refuge for Jenny from the world and her autism, bringing her out of her shell. She could always count on Sparkles to accept her for who she is and to love her unconditionally, which has been for the past fourteen years.

In Memory of Our Mr. Sparkles

Sadly for Jenny, Travis and me, our Mr. Sparkles passed away on March 7, 2015, the day after his fourteenth birthday. We will cherish his memories and will miss him terribly. He brought such joy and sunshine into our lives. He was one in a million and God broke the mould when he made Mr. Sparkles. We can't wait to see you again, Sparks, as we know you will be waiting for us at Rainbow Bridge. We love you, Sparks.

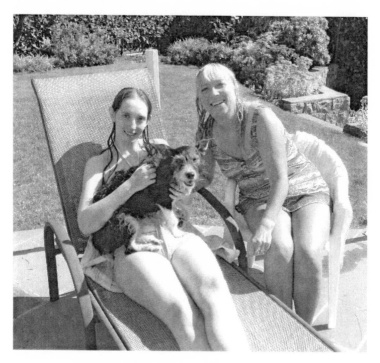

Jenny, Sparkles and I enjoying the sunshine.

Chapter Five

Respite Angels Join the Dream Team

I am so grateful to Dr. Waida for recognizing my need for Respite Care during that first visit after arriving in Vernon. The women who entered our lives in this capacity gave me peace of mind, in addition to providing me with the opportunity to relax, recuperate, breathe, and recharge. Most importantly, however, was the abundance of love, patience, and understanding they showed Jenny as she became a part of their families.

Our Dream Team Grows Further

Margaret Hudson

The first woman I was introduced to was Margaret Hudson, Vernon's Respite Care Co-Ordinator, who arranged for trained individuals to provide respite for parents by caring for their children. We bonded immediately, as it was apparent that Margaret cared deeply for each autistic individual and their family, and would do everything in her power to ensure we received the support we needed. She worked tirelessly the whole time on this and never once wavered.

I took to heart her explanations of why Respite is invaluable for parents, especially when we spend twenty-four hours a day tending to our child's special needs and challenges, all the while participating in workshops and support appointments, in addition to holding down full-time jobs. I also came to the realization that it would be good for Jenny, as it would encourage her to expand her trust circle, while enabling me to be an even stronger support for her.

Once she had collected all our information, Margaret arranged to meet Jenny and assess her needs, so she could match us with the workers best suited to care for her. Her first visit to our home was met with Jenny's usual wariness, complete with spinning in circles and jumping on the couch. Margaret could tell Jenny was disturbed by her presence and tried very hard to remain low key while still taking in what might be required from a caregiver.

Lin Oldfield

The first evidence of Margaret's excellent work was arranging for us to meet Lin Oldfield. Lin came over to our house and I liked her right off the bat. She took to Jenny right away, was very patient with her on this first meeting, and kept her distance so as not to be in her space or upset her. Jenny was jumping up and down on the couch, and then trying to do the same on the coffee table, while I attempted in vain to calm her down. As Jenny displayed her usual anxious behaviour, I was convinced Lin would want to run in the opposite direction. That was not the case at all, however, and Lin offered to be Jenny's and my respite worker.

Lin would visit our home a half-hour at a time initially, so Jenny could get used to her presence with me there for reassurance. It was a slow transition as Jenny grew to trust Lin, but over the course of time they closely bonded to the point that Jenny enjoyed going to Lin's house and spending time with her family. I was eventually able to start leaving her with Lin for longer periods of time—I was incredibly appreciative to have such a sweet and genuine person care for my daughter. Lin started taking Jenny to the movies and out for meals, and they bonded over creativity as Lin is an artist and Jenny loves to draw.

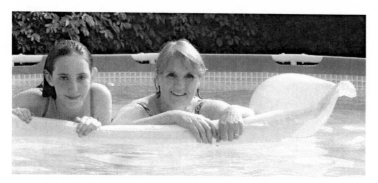

Jenny and Lin have fun in the pool at Lin Oldfield's house.

Chapter Six

Evaluations and Questions Answered

The time had finally come for us to go to Vancouver to have Jenny assessed by a team of specialists, thanks to the waiting list Dr. Waida had placed us on during our initial visit with her. Our appointment with the Vancouver specialists was on October 21, 1997.

As my mother lives in White Rock, Jenny and I drove down on October 20 to stay with her, leaving Chris to stay in Vernon with a friend of his whose family I knew well, ensuring he was able to continue attending school. My mother was there for Jenny and me; however, it was hard for her to see how Jenny acted. She felt so sorry for Jenny and didn't know how to deal with or handle the scenarios that Jenny presented. She would look at me with alarm and uneasiness. I understood and would explain everything to her as situations presented themselves.

One day when we were in a department store in a mall,

the fluorescent lighting started to aggravate Jenny and she launched into a fit. She literally threw herself on the floor and was going red from screaming, hitting, and biting herself. The people around us were horrified, my mother included. Some people were looking at Jenny in disgust and it broke my heart, as they did not understand what this innocent little girl was going through and how many challenges she went through in a day, but I could not just stop going to places and doing things.

I always carried a damp facecloth, in the hopes of cooling her off to settle her. She was so strong, it took every inch of my strength to get her out of the store and back to the car. I remember the whole weekend, my mother saying, "I do not know how you do it. I could not."

She meant well, as she said what a wonderful mother I was and how I was so patient and loving with Jenny in spite of the constant fits and outbursts from the time Jenny woke up to the time she went to bed. I loved Jenny so much and felt that I was her Mama Bear and she was my Baby Bear. I told my mother it was a challenge twenty-four-hours nonstop, that Jenny would have a fit for every change of environment, change of routine, change of food, and every time there were too many people around her. Jenny's five senses were being tested all the time.

I told my mother how fortunate I had been to have met Dr. Waida, because she understood what Jenny was going through and validated my concerns. I explained how grateful I was to her for referring Jenny to the specialists in Vancouver, and how she was instrumental in my agreeing to Respite Care. I reiterated how I wanted to stay strong so I could be there for Jenny and carry on my mission to be her rock, and get her every avenue of care and support. I also mentioned how indescribable it is to explain the hurt when people look at Jenny and talk about her negatively, and how tired I became of explaining her behaviour each time.

It broke my heart to witness Jenny's struggles, but I was determined to be her tank, to boulder through those barriers and set her free from all this. And Jenny herself was such a trooper, fighting to be strong. Her determination was an inspiration to me, and I was learning so much from her.

When my mother heard me say all this and saw my emotions, she gained a greater understanding of what we had been facing, and a new appreciation for what had transpired in the department store.

It was a godsend to be in Vancouver getting Jenny tested and evaluated. We needed to know what was happening with her, and to get help for her right away so we could create a game plan to reach into her world and bring her out. This little girl deserved this.

My mother and I took Jenny for her assessment with a pediatrician, a psychologist, a social worker, and a speech therapist. When they asked me about Jenny, I explained all of her behaviours that we had witnessed, at home and at daycare, being sure not to leave anything out. As they observed her, they saw her demonstrating many behaviours consistent with a diagnosis of autism.

Using a pre-school language scale, they said Jenny demonstrated a severe delay in her understanding of language, her "receptive language development." At that time, Jenny had difficulty comprehending spatial concepts, for example the word *in*. This word and others had little meaning for her.

Testing also revealed Jenny had significant difficulty understanding the use of objects and also pronouns like *they, she, he*. She had difficulty grouping objects, understanding negative phrases, and identifying pictures at her age level. She did not know body parts, and couldn't differentiate between images of animals. Jenny frequently would go to the final words of a phrase or sentence for comprehension, which I had been noticing as well.

They also observed that Jenny had difficulty shifting from one activity to the next—she perseverated with an activity during the assessment and had to be reminded to stop doing what she was doing, to look at her examiner, and to listen to the verbal and visual prompts. Perseveration is the repetition of a particular response, such as repeating a word or phrase, or lacking the ability to transition or switch ideas appropriately within a social context. Even when such a break in activity occurred and a discussion took place reminding Jenny that something new would be required of her, she still perseverated on the previous task.

Throughout the assessment process, I had to ask what some of the medical language meant; knowing these new terms brought me a clearer picture of what was happening with Jenny.

Her receptive vocabulary was restricted for a four-year-old. Jenny demonstrated a severe delay in the development of her expressive language skills—speaking. Tests revealed Jenny had significant difficulty answering questions with yes and no. They revealed she was not yet producing basic sentences of four to five words, and she had significant difficulty explaining how an object is used. She was answering questions without using pronouns; she was unable to discuss remote events. They established through the

"Mean Length of Utterance Test" that her vocabulary was very restricted and her expressive language abilities were severely delayed and disordered.

Jenny also demonstrated disorder in the area of pragmatic development: the ability to deal with things sensibly and realistically. I realize it is good to be pragmatic, but I would have loved her to come out of the black and white area she was always in and into the grey area of spontaneity. They observed that Jenny responded inconsistently to her name and to questions. She would not maintain eye contact with the examiners and would sit with her back to them. She had difficulty with appropriate social skills, saying "Bye, Bye" much later than is considered appropriate. She had odd intonation patterns at times, and exhibited echolalia as well.

Jenny had articulation delay, as revealed by the Goldman-Fristoe Test. She was not positioning a sound normally and would use jargon at times that was unintelligible. I had known at home she was trying hard to communicate, but she understood visual cues better.

Jenny refused to do oral motor tasks during the assessment. They found she could blow bubbles and retract her lips to smile, but she had difficulty pulling her teeth to her bottom lip, and mild difficulty elevating her tongue-tip. She couldn't repeat syllables quickly and with precision. I informed them that Jenny was a very fussy eater but that I had no concerns regarding her ability to chew and swallow food.

Another test they did was the Beery Buktenica Test for visual and motor integration (hand-eye coordination). Jenny was using both hands at this time. However, her left was more dominant. As she got older, her right hand became dominant. Uncannily now she can use the left just as well as the right, but favours the right. At the assessment she was four years and eight months old and she was found to be in the two-year-old range, so she was almost three years behind. The activities in this test—comprising a developmental sequence of geometric designs to be copied with pencil and paper—were very difficult for her.

They gave Jenny the Wechsler Preschool and Primary Scale of Intelligence, which tests general cognitive ability and compares the subject's scores with peers her own age. It involves both verbal and nonverbal skills, as well as listening, organizing, and responding. Jenny tested in the autism range. She couldn't answer questions logically, was unintelligible, and couldn't maintain eye contact. The result was the same with the Verbal Scale IQ and the Performance IQ.

In the Boehm Test of Basic Concepts, Jenny was way behind; some of the concepts she had yet to attain were *nearest, missing, all, around, tallest, backward, finished, lowest, middle, both,* and *outside.*

The next test was the Behaviour Scales, a general assessment of personal and social sufficiency skills conducted with a person who is familiar with the child—in this case—me. The team asked me questions about how Jenny communicated, and about her skills in daily life, socializing, and adapting to change. I told them she had great difficulty understanding concepts and questions. Her understanding of potentially dangerous situations was limited and, consequently, I needed to supervise her closely. At home, she would just run out onto the street; she had no concept of fear, indicated for instance by her use of the playground equipment. I had to be constantly by her side.

Jenny had started to help a wee bit with home chores and she loved to bake with me, with my constant supervision, of course. She was toilet trained, but lots of times during her bowel movements she would run and hide. She was getting better at dressing herself, was slowly starting to observe others at the daycare, and working on social skills. The findings were that Jenny was in the two-year-eight-month age range. Again, she was very behind as she was over four-years-old when this test was done and again this placed her in the Autism/Mild Mental Handicap Range.

The specialists' summary of Jenny at four years old was that she was quiet, had a short attention span, and liked to play with the same toy all the time without changing. Jenny demonstrated a severe receptive language delay and disorder, and had difficulty understanding spatial concepts and the use of objects. She had difficulty in grouping objects, understanding negative phrases, and identifying objects in pictures. It was really hard for her to shift activities, as she tended to perseverate on activities

Ultimately, Jenny had an uneven profile of skills. Her "peaks and troughs" pattern of abilities made learning some tasks very difficult. They said overall her intellectual skills fell within the mild mental handicap range. She exhibited a severe language delay and had problems with planning and coordinating fine motor-skill activities such as copying shapes.

The results of these speech and language tests were consistent with the diagnosis of autism. However at this time, the label "autism" had not been universally accepted, so they had to give her a label of Mild Mental Handicap. We all knew, however, that she was suffering from autism.

They reiterated that we desperately needed a lot of continuous support.

It was emotionally hard for me to hear all this about Jenny; I felt so sorry for her. I wanted to wave a magic wand to make it go away, so she could be like every other four-year-old. I was more than up to the task of finding everything possible to support and help her with all of it. I was a mother on a mission for my child (and you mothers out there know what that means).

So Jenny's slow and uneven development had a label—Mild Mental Handicap; I heard this at the post-assessment conference. I heard that she qualified for services for the mentally handicapped from the Ministry of Children and Family Development. And also that I should continue with respite care as well as obtain access to a childcare worker as Jenny got older.

The registered psychologist recognized all I had been doing to support Jenny and wrote, "Jenny's mother is to be commended for her patience and persistence in attempting to understand Jenny's strengths and weaknesses, and for providing her with a stimulating and supportive environment within which she can be able to develop and progress. It is my impression that Jenny is a much loved little girl who has a very caring Mother and Grandmother. It was a pleasure to meet all three of them."

I left the pediatrician's office, however, in quite a different mood. I had been there for a full day of tests, getting all this overwhelming information, when the pediatrician told me that Jenny would not talk well, and I was basically not to expect her to amount to very much. She said that Jenny would never work in a bank or be able to do math. She went on to say that Jenny would never get married, and there was more, but by this time I was tuning her out.

My mother was tapping my foot as she could see it was

upsetting me and she wanted to help calm me through what this doctor was saying.

I thanked this woman for her time, but as I walked out the door I said, "That is not going to happen."

I was going to do everything in my power to give my girl the world she so deserves. The parent of a child with such handicaps already goes through so much mentally and physically that some are never able to be the rock they need to be. And then to have a doctor saying all this to the parent is like a death sentence for their child's future. I was not at all impressed, and thought, "Even if she means well, that is not how she comes off."

A parent needs someone who really appreciates and understands the situation, and who knows how to handle the scenario with kid gloves and respect, showing some positive light and hope for their child and themselves. Not doom and gloom and, "Well, don't expect much."

I would love to find this woman today and say, "Hello, remember my daughter? Look at her now."

The specialists said that, given Jenny's present development, her progress should be closely monitored and a further psychoeducational assessment should be conducted in the school system in two years. They recommended that Jenny should receive speech and language therapy right away and when she entered the school system. They provided me with advice to give all professionals and the daycare staff who would be working with her. They advised that, prior to giving Jenny verbal instructions, we had to be certain we had her attention through eye contact. This would maximize Jenny's chances of attending to and comprehending questions and commands.

They recommended we give Jenny ample time to respond

to questions, and that we reduce the number of questions we ask at one time—this would reduce her stress level. They explained some facilitation techniques such as labelling common objects, and expanding on Jenny's utterances; in other words, building on what Jenny would say, and then modelling the entire utterance for her. They recommended giving Jenny frequent short breaks to help her maintain her attention during demanding activities.

The team said that Jenny would benefit from access to a teacher assistant and would require assistance to understand instructions, answer questions, and complete activities in her educational settings both at daycare and later in school. Also, she would benefit from communicating with peers her own age. Additionally, they said that supported, cooperative activities with her peers could provide Jenny with situations in which she might confidently learn to interact. They also said that children like Jenny with semantic-pragmatic difficulties tend to benefit from working in small groups. They recommended providing Jenny with opportunities to observe and follow a completed model when teaching her a new skill.

They further suggested using a multisensory approach to teaching concepts, as this would facilitate learning and the retention of new skills. We were to give Jenny additional time to process verbal instructions, formulate her answers, and learn new skills. They said that, in general, Jenny would benefit from an emphasis on visual and contextual cues to facilitate understanding and retention of spoken language.

All the recommendations the team made that day and in written reports were carried out at her daycare, her schools, by all the professionals working with her, and at home. These recommendations and so much more brought Jenny to where she is today.

In addition to receiving these recommendations, I heard that Jenny qualified for services from the Ministry of Children and Family Development. This was like music to my ears and I felt as if we had just struck gold.

I hope by giving readers this information, I am able to offer some insight into the assessment process and thereby enable parents to consider questions and concerns before heading in to speak with the professionals. When we are armed with information, we are in a much better position to support our children.

Chapter Seven

Progress Peeks Through

Jenny's first big breakthrough at daycare occurred when Gail asked her a question and Jenny responded correctly with "a star." This was a huge triumph—generally she would say any word without trying to correlate it to the question asked.

She still resented it when other children wanted to join in her play—she would not let them and would say "Go away" many times and start crying. However, as the year went on I could see that Jenny was saying more words. One day when Shelley was trying to get her to identify pictures, Jenny saw a picture of a witch and said, "I've got you, my pretty." She loved watching the *Wizard of Oz* at home, so she correlated the picture of the witch with the movie. She had also begun making more eye contact.

Over the course of the year from 1996 to 1997, Jenny slowly began to answer more questions appropriately. When asked her name, she understood and knew to respond "Jenny." Her words started to make sense within the context she was using them. I can't describe my emotions the first time she came to the window as I left, and waved to me, saying "Bye, Mum, see you later." I had been praying for this for so long, and I was ecstatic for her.

She was still having sensitivity to noise and large groups of children playing; however, the consistent Theraplay® was yielding results. Jenny was often in a group of five or six children, and most of the time was able to play well, use her words, and make appropriate physical actions. Our goal became to enhance Jenny's self-esteem and increase her trust in others. It gave Jenny positive experiences and let her have fun and healthy social interactions with the other children in the group. We still weren't always clear on what things set her off—she could be so nice one minute, and then turn around and reject everyone around her. This was challenging, and at times I was completely caught off guard when she had a tantrum.

I maintained constant close contact with Darlene, and conferred daily with Shelley, Gail, Deb, and everyone at Brer Rabbit Day Care. I ensured I was active in their group meetings, to help set goals and objectives for Jenny. It meant so much to me that they always included me, letting me be so active and play such a large role in Jenny's itinerary for all the support she was getting. I can't imagine having it any other way, as we all learned so much from each other, and learned even more from Jenny. I discovered how crucial it is for a parent to be included and to stay one hundred and ten percent involved in every aspect of what is going on, ensuring their child's wants and needs are being met.

A major factor in my confidence with Brer Rabbit and our team was the fact that Shelley and the other staff would attend autism workshops on weekends and evenings with me—we all went together. This went so far in showing me they cared and were genuinely invested in the quality of my daughter's life. When I dropped off or picked up Jenny from daycare each day, we were both always greeted with such reassuring happy smiles; over time Jenny's fits began to disappear.

Our team would talk about how Jenny saw the world as black and white—a grey area didn't exist for her. Gail commented that she is the most honest person you could ever meet, as Jenny couldn't understand why people (especially other kids) didn't always do exactly what was asked of them, and it would actually upset her when she witnessed disobedience.

Gail and Deb supplied visual cue cards and posters for Jenny with every type of object imaginable (food items, kitchen utensils, bathroom items, animals, etc.) and she relied heavily on these to respond appropriately. They were so helpful that I made them at home for her too.

It felt like an anvil had been lifted off my chest to see Jenny making advances with her communication. Even with all that the daycare staff was doing, however, it was still an incredibly long process for them, and I appreciated so much their undying patience and constant care for Jenny.

The whole experience really drove home for me how everyone involved in a child's life needs to have a clear understanding of how to accommodate and deal with that child and their behaviour. We need to grab every support system we can and not allow our children to fall through the cracks, or be denied the future and life they so richly deserve. Obviously, navigating autism with our children is very complex and demanding; however, through it all we find a strength that empowers us, breaks down the wall, and reaches out to all who can be there for our child. An early goal is to seek out a qualified pediatrician and specialists.

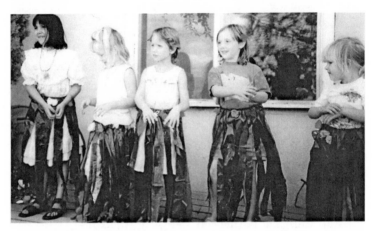

Jenny (second from the right) participates in Hula Dancing.

What Others Shared: Lisa Coley-Donahue, Speech and Language Pathologist

Gradually Jenny warmed to Lisa, and we started seeing dramatic improvements. In a progress report from September, 1997, Lisa mentioned that Jenny was now beginning to use her language in a more spontaneous and appropriate fashion within familiar environments, but that her spoken language was restricted to "here and now" events. Social conversational skills were beginning to emerge but remained limited at this point and Jenny required a "prompter." She was getting the idea of verbal turn taking; however, the content of the information she provided would be inappropriate. For example, when Jenny was asked, "How are you, Jenny?"

Jenny's response could be "My dog is black."

Jenny found it challenging to process the content of what was said and then formulate an appropriate response. This impacted her social interactions. However, her understanding of the concept of positions—*over, under, out, in,* and *through*—had improved. Understanding these helped Jenny express herself better. Some of the goals Lisa was continuing to work on were promoting purposeful play, developing appropriate protesting-and-requesting behaviours, taking turns, and shaping echolalic (repetitive) behaviours into "generative language," by teaching the language rules that children without learning difficulties are able to learn naturally.

"After thirty years of professional practice as a Speech-Language Pathologist, there are some families that stand out in your mind. This is one of those families. When we first met, Janet was desperately seeking help in how best to support her little girl's development. What to do? What to expect? What will the future be like for her? Will she outgrow this? As a community team, we embraced this family. Janet's love for Jenny always shone through no matter what challenging storm brewed. She kept her optimism, humour, and positivity. Hugs, laughter, and always looking ahead kept us moving forward. Janet and Jenny are now living their lives to the fullest. Janet's gift to Jenny has been the unconditional love and support that only a fully engaged parent can give to their child. Thank you, Janet, for sharing your story with us. This is a parent's story that gives us all the gift of hope and the feeling of seeing our children pursue their life passions."

What Others Shared: A Letter From Lin Oldfield, Respite Angel

"I started having respite once a week in Jenny's home. The routine was very similar every week. She liked to have the TV on, even when she wasn't watching it. I went to turn it off one time when she was busy painting, but she quickly got upset, screaming and turning it back on, she liked the white noise. Her painting was interesting too; she only used red paint and she could paint with great ease with a brush in each hand.

"She had a set of Dalmatian Puppy Figurines and she seemed to know exactly how many she had in her hand at one time. If one went missing, we soon knew about it. We had to search the whole house until we found it. She loved lining them up along the bath tub and anywhere else she could find to line them up. I think this must have given her a feeling of order in her very sensorily overloaded young life. Jenny's speech was limited but she could communicate to us when she wanted food or drink by pointing or saying a word that we understood to be milk or cookie.

"Once Jenny was comfortable with me coming to her house and knowing me more, we decided to try doing respite in my home. This turned out to be very successful. We then started doing Respite every other week. And then Jenny came for an actual sleepover. One of the things I remember her doing was to act out the Ariel [*The Little Mermaid*] movie to the soundtrack or DVD. My kids Emma and Dan were fascinated that she seemed to know the entire movie and she went through each scene as if no one else was in the room.

"Routine was crucial for Jenny. When she arrived she discreetly went upstairs to the room where she would be staying and checked I had it in its place. The same with the foods she ate; she liked a limited diet, and I always gave her choices but I knew what she would choose. And when we watched a movie she waited until the movie started before she ate that first piece of popcorn and it lasted until the end of the movie. I guessed that maybe her mum had mentioned at some point that she should wait till the movie started before she started eating and make it last.

"Jenny took most things literally.

"Jenny's manners became incredible. She was very polite in saying please and thank you in all the right places. She knew it was polite to ask people how they were doing when they asked how she was doing and she asked about their day as well. This really impressed me for a young girl who struggled in social settings—she always pushed herself when it must have been awkward for her. Her behaviour was a credit to her mum's hard work.

"It was a pleasure playing a role in Jenny's life, watching her change and grow over the years with all the struggles she had to cope with, and seeing her become such a talented young lady. We shared evenings together sketching or painting or going to the movies or just hanging out. It has been my pleasure."

Lin's comment about the popcorn made me chuckle, as that actually wasn't my doing—Jenny did that on her own!

Lin has lovely memories of Jenny. Lin was then and is still a special person in Jenny's and my lives. Lin took exceptional care of Jenny, and her husband Rob, daughters Emma and Helen, and son Dan were all good to her and great company for Jenny too. I could see the love, care, kindness, and patience Lin always gave Jenny right from the beginning, even when she was such a handful. Lin was always cheerful and accepting of who Jenny was and kept herself mindful of Jenny in every way.

I remember a moment that still gives Lin, Jenny, and

me a good chuckle to this day. I told Lin about how Jenny loved to go to Taco Time® and so Lin would take Jenny there sometimes when she was caring for her. One day, when Lin had her daughter Emma with them and they were enjoying the tacos, Jenny bent over to Emma and quietly said, "You shouldn't talk with your mouth full as you could choke." Lin and Emma looked at each other and Lin said, "You are right, Jenny."

Chapter Eight

Step by Step Jenny Progresses

Once Jenny and I returned home from testing in Vancouver, Margaret Hudson, the Respite Care Coordinator, continued to check in on me to ensure I was still taking full advantage of the Respite Care that was available. We became very close, and would discuss my experiences and what I was learning throughout this process. At one point she actually asked me to talk with the Respite Care workers, offering them insight from a parent's point of view regarding caring for an autistic child. She thought maybe I could share what had worked for Jenny and me, and shed light on additional ways caregivers can support autistic children. I was very happy to oblige, as I had benefitted so greatly from their work and was eager to do anything I could to help them serve their clients.

I remember the first time I started sharing my story about Jenny and her birth—I got a lump in my throat and started to cry. I looked up at all the respite workers listening and discovered they were in tears as well, which I wasn't expecting. The whole experience proved to be quite therapeutic for me, as it was good to revisit the journey and to realize our story could help the workers in how they see and support the children in their care. We discussed a mother's insight, a mother's love, a mother's protectiveness, and a mother's respect and encouragement for her child. It was a real eye opener for us all that evening.

As Jenny got older she started staying overnight at Lin Oldfield's house. I would drop her off around 4:00 p.m. and then Lin would bring her back anywhere between 11:00 a.m. and 1:00 p.m. the next day. Jenny really enjoyed her time at their place as she grew close to all Lin's family. Lin also worked with other autistic and special needs children and teenagers, so she was very aware of how to work with these children and it showed.

By now we had become very close to Gail and Deb from the Brer Rabbit Day Care—they were like our second family. So much so that when Travis and I—we were now engaged to be married—were planning a trip to Hawaii for a week, Gail and Deb looked after Jenny for us. Even though it was hard to leave her and we missed her so much, I knew that I needed this break, relaxation, and some fun, as it had been years since I had done anything without her. Plus, I knew she was in very caring and loving hands.

I can't emphasize enough how grateful we are to these women. They invested one hundred and ten percent of their time, love, and support, and were completely devoted to the children in their care. Whenever I sing their praises they respond so humbly, insisting the work was all on Jenny's and my part, but we could not have found any women more loving to care for Jenny. We credit them as being instrumental in Jenny's rehabilitation from autism—Gail,

Deb, Shelley, and the other staff at "Brer Rabbit" were lights at the end of the tunnel for Jenny.

Respite Angel: Lucy McInnes

As time went on, it became necessary to find a second respite care worker for Jenny for whenever Lin was unavailable. This is when we were introduced to Lucy McInnes. We followed a similar routine for introducing Jenny to new people as we had before, having Lucy visit for short periods of time and taking it slowly. She cautiously and lovingly worked to gain Jenny's trust and let her know she was there for her. She took good care of Jenny, made her laugh, and Jenny felt safe with her. In time, they began doing things together when Lucy came over, and eventually Lucy would take Jenny to her home or out for food or a movie. They spent a lot of time playing games and doing crafts at our house, which Jenny really liked.

Lucy and I became good friends; she was a lovely person to chat with, and was very comedic, always making Jenny and me laugh. She also would be right there whenever we needed her, even on short notice. Lucy meant so much to us, and we so appreciated the love she showed Jenny.

What Others Shared: Lucy McInnes

"I remember going to Janet's home with Margaret and meeting Jenny for the first time. I had a really good talk with Janet, getting to know all about Jenny. I watched her from a distance. However, we had Jenny see me and know I was there, later on. Then I started heading out on a more regular basis to their home and slowly getting to know Jenny and vice versa.

"I found Jenny to be a very shy and sensitive soul. She was not aloof, however. She would be in her room a lot, doing her own thing, being in her own world. I remember her having her own fictional friends, so I didn't want to interfere with that. I let her come to me more, a natural process I used. I wanted to take it slowly with her so she could get to know me on her own timing and terms. I didn't want to upset her and I wanted to make sure we started on the right foot.

"As time went on, Jenny came to trust and accept me and we got along really well. We had a lot of fun times, always having a good laugh or chuckle. By the time I met Jenny, she was no longer having the tantrums or fits; she was around six or seven years old. To this day, I remember Jenny as a very caring, loving, considerate, and kind young girl. She was very considerate of my feelings.

"I remember one time—and Janet and I talked about this recently and chuckled—when Jenny and I were drawing together and I had drawn a duck. After Jenny looked at my duck, I could tell she was wanting to say something about it and was wanting to be kind about it so as not to offend me. She said, 'Lucy, ducks aren't four-legged.' We both looked at the drawing and then at each other and we just started to laugh and couldn't stop. As a matter of fact when I showed the picture to Janet and told her what had happened, she and I laughed so hard we couldn't stop. This is a memory of my time with Jenny and Janet I won't forget.

"Jenny was always a treat to be around, such a sweet personality."

Respite Summary

Even though at first I was reluctant to get Respite, it turned out to be the best thing for both Jenny and me. I was able to go out and do my errands, spend a night out with friends, or do something with my son; and as time went on and I met Travis, we were able to have date nights. I highly recommend for parents of special needs children to take advantage of Respite Care, as it's so important we think of ourselves. We have to remember our children benefit as well, as respite gives us some peace of mind while rejuvenating our mental and physical strength and wellbeing, ensuring our children can depend on us. Additionally, it offers the opportunity for our children to adjust to forming relationships with people outside the family, with the added bonus of those people being trained in the challenges our children face. It really is a win-win situation. Lin (along with her family) and Lucy became great friends to us, and we maintain contact with them to this day.

Furthermore, I was able to meet other families who were in the Respite Care Program, which provided us the opportunity to exchange our life stories and get to know one another and our children. This is vital, because it can be hard parenting a child with special needs—you feel as though no other parent can relate to what you are experiencing. Parents and children would gather at the Christmas parties and other events with the administration and respite care workers and discuss the challenges and the triumphs while the children played games—it was incredibly therapeutic for all involved, and I will always appreciate what they did for us.

Chapter Nine

Kindergarten to Grade 7

Both the Supported Child Care report and the examination reports from the specialists in Vancouver made it clear that when going into kindergarten Jenny would require supported education and special assistance. She would have her special assistant at times in the actual classroom, and then would leave the classroom and spend learning time in the Learning Assistant's Room. In 1998 and 1999, a plan and an assessment were done, stating that the main areas Jenny would require assistance with were language and concept development. Social skills were another important area that she would require support in, to develop her socialization skills and to play interactively with her peers. Finally, the next support required was in the area of Independence Skills, such as self-care, making choices, and following directions.

I made sure I was apprised of what Jenny's daily schedule and learning would entail when she entered kindergarten. This was a huge change of routine for Jenny, from being at home and at Brer Rabbit for the last couple of years to a whole new environment with lots of new people. A crucial step in this transition came when the school had the kindergarten teacher come to our home in June 1998, so she could introduce herself to Jenny, Travis, and me before kindergarten started in September. Jenny acted up as she knew there was a strange presence in her midst. I have a photograph of her being held by Travis that day, with her blanket clutched strongly in her hand as she didn't want to stay in the room with this stranger. Travis was gently trying to get her to stay and so he held her. This visit offered insight to the teacher as to how Jenny would be in need of assistance in her class.

What Others Shared: Brer Rabbit Day Care

Brer Rabbit Day Care only went to a certain age so it was terribly sad to leave there as they had been so wonderful, and Jenny had made such strides in improving her socialization skills with the children there, because she was comfortable. It was hard for Gail and Deb too, as Jenny had become such a special little girl in their lives.

Jenny received a letter from Gail, Deb, and the girls at Brer Rabbit when she set off for kindergarten.

"Jenny, we started in June 1996 on a journey together, with a mother's prayer, 'If only my child could tell me about her day.' Jenny you were a child unable to communicate your basic needs. Antisocial, unaware of the world around you. Wow, look at you now. The changes are spectacular, Jenny.

"We liken you to a sponge as you seemed to absorb and immerse yourself in your topic to experience and discover everything there is to know about this subject. Jenny, you have a flair for the theatrical, like the famous actress your mother is. You have a love of music, dance, and chocolate. You are outstanding as a puppeteer. You enjoy videos, colouring, animals, computer games, and storybooks. You're determined, strong-willed, and compassionate about those you love. You have very strong likes and dislikes.

"This year, you have been willing to try new foods—way to go! You are smart, creative, adventurous, and physically strong. Playful, with a great sense of humour, and persistent, you enjoy structure and seem confident as a leader. Jenny, you have made incredible strides in your speech. You are truly alive in this world. Thank you for including us in your journey as it has been great. We learned so much from you and we know you will do really well in kindergarten."

When September rolled around, I remember taking a deep breath and saying, "Here we go—Jenny's first day of school!" I was overcome with emotions that ran the gamut from sadness at seeing her grow up, to excitement for the new journey ahead, to concern over how she would adjust to all the changes, while wondering whether she would be accepted by her peers.

Jenny attended Okanagan Landing School, which was pretty close to our home. The primary goal in the beginning (both for us her family at home and the teachers and staff at the school) was to ensure Jenny was comfortable with the routines and behaviour expectations placed on her in the classroom. The staff did this by giving her verbal warnings in class and a quiet reminder to her as needed before a schedule change.

I really appreciated that the school stressed the importance of a schedule for Jenny—it was set out each morning before school began, to reinforce activities for her. Visual pictures and cards were big learning tools for her in school, as words and sentences were hard for her. One big goal we all had for Jenny was increasing her knowledge and use of basic language concepts, for example *in, off, under, out of, together, happy versus sad, soft versus hard, heavy versus light, fast versus slow.*

The next goal (and of primary importance to me) was her socialization and interaction with peers. Her Certified Education Assistant and Special Learning Personnel used strategies of modelling and role playing with her. They did guided play and scripted routines, which helped Jenny to greet her peers with appropriate phrases like "Hello" and "Good morning." We hoped to see Jenny begin to initiate conversations with her peers.

Jenny also needed support with the development of emergent literacy skills, so they used story maps and props to help her with this. Items were labelled with their names and functions. They used visual word vocabulary cards to assist her everyday language development and also in sequence for retelling events and well-known stories. Repetition was key to success in her learning. A directed activity would be scaled down to her level and, even though she might not comprehend the big picture, it would still work at her level.

On completion of Jenny's year in kindergarten in 1999,

her teacher Mrs. Corbett told me that Jenny had made significant progress through the year. Mrs. Corbett was pleased with Jenny's gains in expressive language, but said that although Jenny worked very hard, she still had a serious language delay. Apparently, Jenny would go two steps forward and then one back.

With Mrs. Corbett saying this, I made sure to continue to read stories to Jenny on a daily basis, which I loved doing. After reading the story, we would talk about it together. I also would encourage Jenny to practise her writing with her current knowledge of letters and spell them out in messages. Jenny and I would review one letter name and sound it out, in the same way it was being taught in her animated alphabet lessons in kindergarten class. Also incorporated into our home routines, I would teach her counting; for the concept of the number four, we would count out four cookies, four pieces of bread, or four carrots. We played a lot of board games, which we loved doing together and in turn this would reinforce number recognition and provide meaningful counting practice—and make it fun, too.

In May 2000, Jenny had her next session with Dr. Pipher. His follow-up report stated that Jenny continued to struggle with language deficits, had few friends at school, and continued to experience extreme difficulties labelling emotions. In addition, she was prone to anxiety.

I let him know that Jenny was participating in a Therapeutic Horse Riding Program and he felt that would be very helpful for her—both for her social skills as well as her gross motor skills and balance development. Jenny really enjoyed riding the horse and I felt it assisted her with her autism. I was sad when the program stopped due to cost cuts, as it was so therapeutic and mind opening for her.

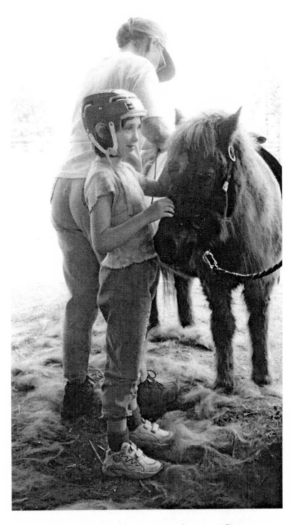

Jenny attends therapeutic horse riding.

Dr. Pipher recommended that Jenny continue with speech language therapy, which we did. I agreed with everything he said as she still was having problems in talking with her peers, and knowing how to converse and play with them—she didn't know how or want to initiate play.

Mrs. MacDonald, Jenny's teacher for Grade 1 in 2000, felt that Jenny made a good adjustment from half-day schooling to a full day, and that she had a positive attitude and made good effort toward her school work. Mrs. MacDonald told me that Jenny excelled when it came to art activities and that she also enjoyed class singing times and poetry reading. She said Jenny was able to "read" the poems and songs from memory. She had two main areas of focus for Jenny: blending letter sounds together to form them into words in her journal and gaining confidence for sharing ideas in class discussions. Mrs. MacDonald said she found Jenny lacked the confidence to believe in herself.

During the time that Jenny was in Grade 1, I continued to review songs, poem sheets, and reading books daily at home with Jenny. We would practise her writing skills by having her help me with a grocery list or doing cards and letters for family members. We would practise counting and printing numbers as well by 2's, 5's, and 10's up to 100.

Jenny had Mrs. MacDonald again the following year in 2001 for Grade 2; it was a Grade 1/2 split class. Jenny was still working on her Grade 1 learning outcomes, which she reached that following year. Her vocabulary had increased, though she still guessed a lot of words as she had little to no ability with phonics. Jenny was receiving learning assistance for reading, writing, and math skills. She couldn't yet formulate a story with a beginning, a middle, and an end, but her skills were developing. Mrs. MacDonald told me that Jenny continued to work below the level expected for her age.

I kept up the reading at home every day and continued to help Jenny write letters to family and friends, even starting a journal with both letters and drawings. I always made it fun, and we played games with dice and card games to work on her addition and subtraction skills.

Kid Zone

While Jenny was in Elementary School, we needed to find her an after-school daycare. I dreaded starting out all over again with a new environment—new faces, new kids—this was definitely going to be disruptive for Jenny. I was praying we would find a place like Brer Rabbit.

I did my research and found an after-school daycare on the same grounds as Okanagan School. I made an appointment with Kid Zone and met the lovely Carmen Laferriere. We researched together to make sure that their setting would meet the goals and criteria for Jenny's needs. They did have some children with special needs, but these children had no support or special caregivers with them, which unfortunately would not work in Jenny's scenario.

Carmen was concerned at first as the facility would need to hire extra staff for Jenny. It would be extremely difficult to assist Jenny in developing her social skills and language without a one-on-one assistant on a daily basis. Carmen and I pushed for this and asked for a Special Certified Caregiver to continue to help Jenny develop a strong foundation for her language and social skills. The reports from all the medical and psychological professionals who worked with Jenny showed she required this level of care, and we explained that without an assistant she would continue to withdraw from social interaction and revert back to old behaviours.

We wanted continuity in the work being done at her school to carry on to her daycare support as well. This meant the person working with Jenny at Kid Zone would implement the peer interaction program based on Michael Guralnick's "Peer Interaction Model." Also we needed the language goals identified by the school therapist to be supported appropriately. All of this meant an extra staff member would be needed. Kid Zone and I asked Supported Child Care for a four-hour position five days a week for the first twelve weeks, to be reviewed before Christmas. Happily we got this for the entire time Jenny was at Kid Zone, until funding ran out for the facility itself and it was closed down entirely. In the time she was there, however, the staff and I saw changes in Jenny from her first step through the door to her last day.

The first report Kid Zone provided highlighted how Jenny was sensitive to external stimuli. It also stated she was very much routinized, so if there was any change in the schedule she needed to know ahead of time and to understand why—otherwise it would throw her off and she would have crying sessions or fits. Once she understood the routines and expectations, however, she would participate positively.

The people who worked with Jenny at Kid Zone were very patient, caring, loving, and understanding with her. Jenny was starting to be able to wash and dress herself at this time. However, she was not good with matching colours and designs together so I would help her out with that. She had difficulty tying her shoelaces and would rather wear shoes with Velcro® or ones that didn't have ties as they were easier for her. They saw that Jenny needed support in social settings as they found she tended to often play on her own. In time, she began to interact better with her peers, though they found she preferred to play with children younger than herself. As Jenny was a couple of years behind developmentally, it seemed appropriate that she did this.

As for playing at Kid Zone, she loved swimming and drawing and playing on the computer. She loved to read books and she loved animals. She seemed to enjoy music, singing, and dancing. She enjoyed art, dress-up, bubbles, ball games, and outdoor play. However, she still preferred to play on her own and in small groups.

Jenny had a tendency to talk with a high-pitched baby voice. So at Kid Zone and at home we would say, "Use your 'big-girl' voice." To this day, Jenny has a unique sweet tone to her voice. It is still childlike and very quiet. Kid Zone staff said Jenny was always requiring extra time to respond, and if she was rushed or didn't understand she would say, "I don't know."

Jenny could solve simple problems and recognize whole words. However, she had difficulty with phonetics. She still had a one-and-a-half to two-year delay in her development. The daycare followed naturally occurring opportunities for her learning. They found her to be a bit clumsy so she needed to improve her fine motor skills. They found Jenny sensitive and high-strung. They also saw that Jenny was a "black and white" thinker. When Jenny was holding something in, she would withdraw and become anxious. She knew her limits and understood what others should do. They also pointed out that Jenny was a good-natured girl.

In Kid Zone's second report dated September 17, 2000,

staff reported that Jenny required pre-warnings for what was coming up and would get quite distressed if she did not know what was going on. She became withdrawn, and when the group was loud and fast paced she would find a place to be on her own. For snacks she had specific dislikes of certain food, which appeared to correlate with texture. They noticed that while she was still playing alone she watched quite closely what others were playing with and then would move closer to play alongside them. She played cooperatively with one boy and would often reject others' attempts to join her in play. She would use a small voice and tell them "No" or to leave, as well as hiding toys with her body. When Jenny got hurt emotionally, she would cry and withdraw, but not seek adult help—consequently the adults needed to be able to predict when this might occur.

In her play, activities, and interests, Jenny liked to manipulate things and arrange them. She enjoyed computers and music paired with movement. She observed other children playing house. Board games drew her interest and she liked to play with balls. In communicating, she was more likely to respond positively if someone made eye contact first and were positioned close to her. Loud ambient noise made it more difficult for her to follow verbal directions and, when peers made requests of Jenny, she would become anxious—so daycare staff felt she needed simpler language.

The fast pace of Kid Zone seemed to affect her anxiety level and when she tried to assert herself the other children didn't hear or understand her. When a novel situation occurred Jenny would like to be part of the group. However, she would need adult prompting, assurance, or direct help. The staff were concerned that Jenny didn't have the skills to deal with confrontations or novel problems in an effective manner. This especially was a concern of mine as she couldn't defend herself appropriately. When they went bowling or did other activities, she needed coaxing to participate and initially didn't want to go.

The workers at Kid Zone were fantastic with Jenny, and I cannot sing high-enough praises for Carmen and Mel Price, Jenny's one-on-one workers. They were loving, caring, and genuinely wanted Jenny to succeed and achieve her life goals. We would have meetings together and exchange information about Jenny in terms of her socialization, communication, conversation, and peer play. We would share any concrete results on different strategies that were working with her, and brainstorm about new approaches. I was very sad when Kid Zone closed their doors because of money cuts. They were an amazing group of people and Jenny was slowly making friendships there—really starting to thrive and do well. Jenny and I are still in contact with Mel, as she is a sweetheart and a wonderful woman.

What Others Shared: Mel Price-Ouellette—Kid Zone

"What stands out in my memory about you and Jenny is your close relationship with each other. Your dedication toward wanting and succeeding in making Jenny's life extraordinary was very evident. I remember Jenny was a little sweetie and I loved my time at Kid Zone; you both felt like family to me."

Our next follow up with Dr. Pipher was in April 2001. He stated that Jenny's language remained poor but that she was showing signs of improvement. Slowly but surely we could see her vocabulary expanding. He was happy to hear that Jenny was receiving assistance as he considered it very important for her mental and physical wellbeing and her future. He and I talked about Jenny being a couple of years behind mentally, and how she preferred to play with children younger than herself. He noticed, as did I, that Jenny was still sensitive and prone to anxiety. He also noted her sensitivity to change and uncertainty. She still had some overpowering tantrums, but they were becoming less frequent and severe, so this was promising. He also drove home the need for a Psychoeducational Assessment, as Jenny was a child with unique needs.

The School District did a Psychological Assessment of Jenny in November 2001. We wanted to ensure she would be receiving as much support as possible both in and outside school. At the beginning of her assessment, the school psychologist noted that Jenny initially demonstrated some reluctance to participate in the process. The psychologist spent time trying to suppress Jenny's anxiety by having her draw, which Jenny always loved. Then she asked what Jenny liked to do at school. The assessment didn't start until Jenny began to demonstrate a more relaxed behaviour; however, the psychologist felt that Jenny never became completely comfortable during the process. Jenny participated to the best of her ability, though, and it was considered a valid assessment of her intellectual capabilities.

The first test was the Wechsler Intelligence Scale for Children, used to establish Jenny's abilities in intelligence and verbal ability and performance. The psychologist found Jenny to be in the mild mental handicap range, falling into the 0.1 percentile. She demonstrated severe language deficits, which interfered with her ability to comprehend and to interpret language. A reflection of severe receptive language delay contributed to her limitation with verbal intellectual capabilities.

The next test was the Performance Scale IQ, which provides information about the ability to interpret visual images and to form abstract concepts without the use of words. Jenny demonstrated strength in her visual ability to perceive, organize, and identify solutions to concrete problems. Jenny's score suggested that her strengths lie in her nonverbal abilities, and this indicated that a significant discrepancy existed between her verbal and nonverbal abilities.

With Jenny having the type of profile she has, she had difficulty learning school-related tasks. The psychologist told me Jenny's academic progress would continue to be slow and her development would continue to be significantly less than children of average ability.

She explained that a child with this type of profile would find the school environment very frustrating without the appropriate intervention. Fortunately, Jenny wasn't showing or experiencing severe behaviour problems within the school setting at this time, which indicated the school was able to accommodate the weakness effectively.

Jenny's high performance on picture completion, picture arrangements, block designs, and object assembly subtests indicated these to be areas of strength for her. She could tell the difference between things. For instance, she could see that the round block fitted in the round hole, where the square one would not.

In summary, these results were along the lines of the autism, with Jenny having a mild mental handicap. The psychologist told me that, with her type of profile, Jenny would continue to require individual educational programming to best meet the special needs due to her autism.

Then the psychologist discussed the area I was primarily concerned with—social situations. She said it would become increasingly difficult for Jenny to cope as her peers become more proficient language users. She told me that to limit Jenny's frustrations, she needed pre-teaching strategies for new situations. These would require a group effort between me and the school. I left that session determined to ensure Jenny continued receiving the support she required.

For Grade 3 in 2002, Jenny had Miss Desmarais. She was a true blessing for Jenny in Elementary School, a sweetheart and a lovely person. Jenny really liked her and she was very engaging and patient with Jenny. Miss Desmarais took time to understand Jenny and to be there for her the whole year through. She felt Jenny enjoyed some successes that school year and said that Jenny worked very hard, made steady gains, was responsible for her homework, and tackled her home reading with diligence. Also, Jenny should be proud of herself for having read so many books. Miss Desmarais commended Jenny for her persistence to improve, which helped Jenny gain some confidence as a learner. Jenny did well in making the transition to handwriting with some good results. However, I will personally say to this day Jenny hates handwriting and would rather print any day than write. Even when it comes to forms she has to sign, she will ask me, "Can't I print?"

In Jenny's Grade 3, the Learning Assistance teacher, Shawna Buffie, said they had seen a growth in Jenny—she had more confidence in herself and was able to read Grade

2 material with more confidence. However, if a new word came along, she would freeze. When Jenny was asked to talk about what she had read, she would remember some details, but miss others, which then made it difficult for her to make conclusions as to why things had happened. Jenny also needed help with counting money and understanding the concept of time. She found Jenny pleasant to work with and said she was nice to other students.

At home we continued to read, journal, and play games all year long. I made the reading sessions short and fun and we would always talk about the story with questions for her to answer. When we went to the store I had Jenny count out money to give to the cashier. She would get shy though, so that was harder for her. She could tell the time at the half hour and hour, but could not understand the fifteen-minute intervals.

Jenny's school and I worked actively together to contribute to positive experiences for her. I pushed hard for her special needs help through an assistant aid. I was always in touch with this person as well as with Jenny's teacher and principal. I can't stress enough how vital it is for us parents to fight for the support our children require, as I saw another mother not get the support and guidance that Jenny and I had, and I found it very sad that she and her child went through a lot of issues because of their lack of support.

Jenny had an exceptional group of teachers, assistant aids, and special resource teachers in her seven years at Okanagan Landing. Each year from Kindergarten to Grade 7, her individual teachers and aids were always respectful and immersed themselves in what Jenny required, whether it be of an academic or social nature.

From Grades 4 through 7, Jenny's teachers worked on improving her math skills. The expectations in math were scaled back so that she was not required to produce at the level of the regular program students. They felt her math was at a Grade 3 or 4 level in Grade 6.

Jenny used simple vocabulary and sentence structure to write short pieces independently that dealt with familiar topics. One of her teachers was Mr. Cecile and he said Jenny enjoyed writing in the classroom. She still liked to read simple chapter books, but with support she was able to do novel study activities. When reading independently, Jenny would miss important details. I noticed at home that she seemed to only pick up some of a sentence when reading. So her ability to decode was still stronger than her ability to comprehend, especially with non-fiction pieces.

One thing that I stressed to the teachers and learning assistants during these grades was her social skills. The friends Jenny had at this time were able to adjust themselves to her interests. In time, she was able to converse a bit better with her peers, but when she was conversing with adults, the teachers had to work to keep the dialogue going. This changed as she got older and actually reversed so that she conversed better and more comfortably with the adult teachers in high school than with her peers.

During these last few years of elementary school, I had Jenny read books to me and, after each chapter, I would have her relate to me what she thought about it and give me some details. When she came shopping with me I would have her help count out the money or look at the receipts and make sure the totals were right. We would go to events that required socializing and meeting people—both children and adults—to get Jenny feeling comfortable with conversing.

Jenny had both good and bad moments through these years. At times, she would get frustrated and act out, or shut down and go on her own to break down and cry. There were also several occasions she would come to the car crying because someone had teased her, or she felt no one was listening or understanding her.

I always felt bad for Jenny as I know that during a lot of these early school years she kept to herself and didn't make friends because of her language barrier, social issues, shyness, and being in her own world. Other children would look at her and think she was strange, different, and very quiet. She knew how they felt and looked at her—that she was different and didn't belong. She liked to take her "blankie" to school for the first couple of years, as it would help her cope—but because of it, she would get teased and made fun of.

Jenny did make two good friends during this time, however. Mercedes and Noelle lived on the same block as us and she played with them from six years old to around ten years old. They were two to three years younger than her, but, considering where she was developmentally, they got along really well, and it gave us hope that Jenny was learning how to socialize.

At school functions, however, Jenny was always very quiet—not saying much and just looking around—I could tell she was anxious and nervous. In her first few years at events we attended with her, Jenny stuck close by Travis and me, and just watched what the other children were doing. It was heartbreaking to witness, as I wished her peers would be more understanding of who she was and not just look past her.

We attended another follow-up session with Dr. Pipher

in 2002, when Jenny was nine years old. He observed that there were still significant expressive and receptive language disorders and mental challenges, and that she was still shy, anxious, and easily agitated. He felt that from what he was hearing from me, the daycare, and the professionals who were working with her, Jenny's ability to socialize was slowly improving. We still had to work on encouraging her to become assertive for herself with others, instead of retreating inside herself and crying. Dr. Pipher stressed that the extra support for Jenny—both at school and during after-school care—had to be ongoing. He stressed the same for the speech and language therapy.

At this time I decided to retire from working as a dental assistant and hygienist after twenty-seven years and I actually found a job where we ended up not needing daycare. Between Travis's, my son's, and my work schedules, one of us could always take Jenny to school while another could always pick her up.

We next visited Dr. Pipher in June 2003, when Jenny was ten years old. I made him aware that Jenny was becoming more comfortable in the classroom setting but still had quite a way to go. She appeared to be managing better, thanks to the extra support at school, and was slowly developing relationships with peers her own age. I informed him that Jenny left regular classes to visit the Learning Centre for help with language and concept development, social skills for play and conversation, and independent skills for self-care and making choices. He was happy to hear about all this and said that, even though she still had the language disorder and intellectual challenges, she was now able to provide some logical rationale, which was incredibly promising.

Jenny made a couple of friends later on in Elementary School, one of whom was Lisa Rae, who's been an absolute blessing in Jenny's life. Lisa understood her best, and is still a very good friend to Jenny. She has always understood Jenny and accepted her for who she is, never judging her. I believe she has been incredibly helpful in assisting Jenny to socialize, as Jenny feels very comfortable with her. Lisa is someone Jenny could talk with in her own way, and still feel understood.

I always had birthday parties for Jenny through these elementary school years and invited other girls from her classes in the hopes they would befriend Jenny. She was only ever invited to one in return, however. I always felt for Jenny in this regard, but all I could do was try.

In 2005, we had our last follow-up appointment with Dr. Pipher, when Jenny was twelve years old. He informed me that in his opinion Jenny would suffer from a life-long disability, and that her emotional, social, and behavioural needs would require special assistance for the rest of her school years. Dr. Pipher had guided Jenny through many avenues of her development, and it was a pleasure talking with him about Jenny on each visit.

I know Jenny's differences bothered her a lot as she got older, as she felt like she didn't belong and that no one liked her. It wasn't that she necessarily wanted to be "Miss Popular," but just to fit in, be able to have fun, converse, and relate with the other students. I saw a glimmer of hope at her Grade 7 grad party, though. She was with Lisa and Jewel , and was walking around with them and a few others, playing games, and dancing—she was actually enjoying herself! Later she confided to me that she had felt very nervous and unsure, but I told her she should be proud of herself, as that took a lot of courage.

Chapter Nine

What Others Shared: Lisa Rae-Babchuk

"Jenny is my best friend. We went to the same elementary school and I actually met her when I was two years old. We got to know each other more when we were in Grade 5. We were in separate classes but I started to hang out with a girl Jenny knew. Jenny was shy but honest and a lot of fun. She liked to run around and be silly. She never played mind games like other kids did. She and I had the same attitude about having fun and knew that there would be time to grow up in high school. I didn't have many friends in elementary school and I am really glad I got to know Jenny.

"Jenny has always been shy and quiet. There have been times where she's just trying to ask me a question like, 'What time is it?' and I can't hear her. I'd ask her to speak up, but it would come out the same volume. We would just laugh when this happened because it would be the silliest thing but I just couldn't hear her. As we grow, I see Jenny as more private than shy. She is the type of person who gets to know people slowly. Jenny is honest about who she is and what she likes; she doesn't play social games that most people do. I remember Jenny sometimes asking if it was okay to like something, like a song or a book, but then just as many times she would say how much she liked something and didn't care if it was cool or not."

What Others Shared: Jackson Mace—Jenny's Teacher in Grades 4 and 6

"I remember Jenny so very well! Not because she was the most scholastic student I've ever taught, but rather for reasons that only a teacher could cherish. I remember her bright and warm smile; a smile that shone like the Aquila at the slightest bit of humour or praise. I remember her work ethic and the bond she had with her mother and my friend, Janet; their determination to get things right! I remember the sense of pride as she attached herself to all she attempted, especially when an opportunity arose to display her natural talent for drawing. But most of all, I remember a young lady who took what she had and did the best she possibly could with it, day after day after day. That was Jenny and those qualities are enduring and memorable."

I looked up the word *Aquila*: it is a constellation that is shaped like an eagle and has one very bright star.

What Others Shared: Shawna Buffie—Grade 4 Teacher and Learning Assistant

"Jenny is a very pleasant student who has made substantial progress during her school years. She has been on an Individual Education Plan and receives support through our Learning Centre. Jenny's goal areas include building skills in reading, math, oral language, social skills, and fine motor ability. Jenny's progress has been steady and we are very pleased with her gains in all these areas.

"Jenny continues to have difficulty with phonetic activities but her strong visual skills enable her to memorize new sight words daily. Language goals developed with the input of the Speech Language Pathologist continue to be worked on informally in the classroom and small groups. Jenny is working, in particular, on sequencing activities and using the appropriate language to retell stories and events. Jenny's fine motor ability has improved as well, and she draws and colours beautifully.

"Jenny can be a shy little girl but we have seen a noticeable growth in her self-confidence. Jenny used to have episodes where she would become 'weepy' and upset. These incidents have decreased and she is happy and compliant most of the time. Jenny responds best when her day and her activities are structured and predictable.

"It is clear that Jenny is very well supported at home and that her mother and stepfather work very hard to enrich her learning experiences. I, as well as the other teachers working with Jenny, am in frequent contact with Jenny's mother, Janet, and I appreciate her caring and enthusiastic attitude toward Jenny's learning. We feel that Jenny is a very well-supported child and that she will continue to move forward as long as this support system remains in place."

Chapter Ten

High School Years—The First Half

In September, 2006, Jenny headed into Grade 8 at Clarence Fulton High School. I watched her march into Fulton on her first day alongside over nine hundred other students and I knew she was anxious—this wasn't going to be easy for her.

We had visited Fulton in June 2006 while Jenny had still been in Grade 7 at Okanagan, so that the Special Education Teachers could meet with Jenny before school started and get to know her. We wanted to have everything planned for what she would be needing while attending school there. Wendy Goodall from Okanagan Landing was the individual who was responsible for making the appointment at Fulton and making Jenny's move from elementary school to high school as smooth and comfortable as possible.

We met up with Lisa Devana Balcombe at Fulton, who was Jenny's case manager for her transition. That day, Jenny learned the layout of the school building and locations of various places such as the administration office, her locker, the washrooms, cafeteria, and the games rooms. Her placement for subjects was to be in a regular program in all areas except for Adjusted Math 8. She was to be placed in regular classes with her friend Lisa Rae whenever possible. Jenny was not to be given two academic subjects per day, and was to be connected with an adult who would mentor her and check in with her on a regular basis. We were hoping this would help with her transition.

The Individualized Education Plan for Jenny's initiation to Grade 8 listed five goals. They all centred on objectives, strategies, support, and personal adjustments. She was to receive direct classroom instruction and extra support from a Certified Education Assistant and a Learning Aids Teacher. They would review instructions to make sure she was understanding what was asked of her, and then break the information up into steps that would allow her more time to process the information. The length of her assignments was also adjusted to lower the difficulty of the material.

Jenny's homework completion and progress were also monitored. The Certified Education Assistant helped her with writing effectively to communicate what she knew or had learned and to write proper sentences, using correct capitalization, punctuation, and grammar. Jenny was to practise this by writing a simple short story with a beginning, a middle, and an end. They then collected and analyzed her writing samples and assessed them under the Wechsler Individual Achievement Test.

Lisa and the Certified Education Assistant wanted to improve Jenny's PM Benchmark—a tool that tests a child's reading age—from a Grade 3 to a Grade 4 Level. In doing this they were teaching Jenny to learn strategies to decode new and unfamiliar words and to self-correct when a word didn't make sense. They would always check with me that she was reading at home, and I was pleased to report that she was actually enjoying reading. She would come to me and ask about a word, sentence, or paragraph when she didn't understand. Assessments were done throughout the year, and her teachers would assist in monitoring her improvement.

The most important goals in my eyes were in the areas of social, emotional, and behavioural development. The overall objective was to help Jenny develop her social skills, as this is an area that made her quite anxious; we hoped to see her develop and maintain friendships with peers her age. Jenny's classroom teacher was to role model appropriate social skills, and to support and encourage her to make friends. Jenny would also do small group practice with the Certified Education Assistant to increase her participation in class.

Jenny went above and beyond all these goals in a shorter period of time than anticipated, much to the excitement and happiness of everyone at the school and her family. She did not require the special help for very long and wanted to go out on her own, which astounded everyone. However, the goals she continued to struggle with were social skills. Her self-esteem fluctuated wildly and I had to work on it with her every day. I'm sure a lot of her teachers and some students didn't even notice, but for Jenny, every day was a social challenge, and often resulted in tears.

Lisa, Jenny's Case Manager, had been told Jenny came with a label, and though she agreed that Jenny didn't talk much, she maintained that Jenny listened very well.

Lisa said when Jenny spoke, she spoke with purpose and wisdom, choosing her words carefully. She also said that Jenny took a different path—not the one expected; she would choose her path carefully, always keeping her final destination in mind. Even when the path appeared to be too steep or treacherous, Jenny forged on.

One perspective that Lisa shared about Jenny—one that is my favourite—was that she thought the label should have said, "The best is yet to come." Lisa added that she was very thankful to have known Jenny and that Jenny reminds her every day that "a story is not written until the author writes it, and Jenny is a great writer."

Jenny ended up receiving Honour Roll Standing in Grade 8, but even having conquered such odds, she still came to the car many days crying, upset, and feeling awful. I would hug her so hard, wipe her tears, and tell her what a wonderful girl she was—that the other kids didn't know what they were missing in not befriending her. I can't imagine going up against all the challenges high school presents in addition to having special needs.

Jenny worked very hard in both her regular and special classes, and I enjoyed reading the teachers' comments in her school reports, as they not only demonstrated who Jenny was as a student, but also who she is as a person. I would show these to Jenny to give her insight on what people thought of her and to boost her self-esteem. She would smile and be so humble about it ... this is why it would pain me so much that she would experience bullying, and that her peers were not warming up to her.

In her first year at high school she had to switch lockers as the boy at the next locker would constantly tell her she was ugly and stupid. When she tried to get into her locker, he would stand in front of it and refuse to move. Another boy refused to hit the volleyball when she served—acting as though it had germs—she said he made her feel so ugly. During dodgeball practice, he would throw the ball hard, right at her chest, and would mock anything she said, saying it was stupid and giving her dirty looks. Yet another boy would criticize and laugh at her art work, and constantly poke her. This type of behaviour must have been unbearable, as she was under so much pressure as it was, but she was a lot stronger than she realized to keep soldiering on in school.

She would become very frustrated, because often when she wanted to stick up for herself, she couldn't figure out what to say until it was too late. I thank God for Lisa, Cierra, and a couple of other girls who befriended her during this time. Jenny actually felt like she fit in with them, and was "heard." Jenny's language and conversation barrier would often pull her deeper inside herself, as she so badly wanted to say things correctly and not sound stupid. Jenny was into art and animation but not much else, so she found it hard to participate in conversations on other topics. When she did try, the students would often just ignore her and, though she had a few friends, they had full lives, which resulted in Jenny feeling very alone at times.

On the academic front, Jenny worked extremely hard and achieved the highest marks in her math class. When we heard that news, I told her about her assessment back when she was a little girl and how they proclaimed she would never succeed in math. I made sure to drive home to her how proud I was of her for proving them wrong. I think that was the first time I actually saw Jenny feel pride in herself, and it is a cherished moment for me to look back on.

Jenny's Grade 8 English teacher, Mrs. Woodliffe, told me that Jenny met all expectations with her marks throughout the entire course, and her final exam score indicated she had mastered many of the major concepts covered that year. This was incredible news, as Jenny had required no adaptions or special help in this course, and was achieving these heights on her own. Step by step, things were looking up and the hard work she was investing in herself was paying off.

What Others Shared: Cierra Carlyle

Cierra Carlyle is one student who saw Jenny for who she is. Cierra, who just came to visit Jenny recently, shared some memories of meeting her in high school.

"I remember the very first time I met Jenny. We were in English 8 and were asked to team up with classmates to practise for a spelling test. A new friend of mine invited Jenny to our group because she was sitting close to us. She seemed quiet and shy and very nervous in her speech. It didn't bother me at all. Why would I judge someone I had just met? That shy and nervous girl quickly became one of my best friends. It wasn't until a few months into our friendship that Jenny opened up to me and told me she had autism. She thought I would treat her differently ... like so many people had before. To me, she was still the same, beautiful, compassionate, and funny person, but I [then] became much more aware of the issues she had to face every single day.

"Reading, math, writing, and being in large groups were just some of the things she would tell me about that she struggled with…. The thing I admired the most about Jenny was her work ethic. Even though things were hard and would take a lot of extra effort to do, she would do them and do an outstanding job. Through high school, I watched her go through a lot. One of the biggest struggles was bullying. From people turning and laughing at her in class to someone who Jenny thought was a good friend cyberbullying her. I still cannot believe how much she had to endure, but I am so glad she had a good group of friends to support her and show her that no matter what someone says, you are better than the words they say."

Jenny's good friend Lisa remained her biggest supporter through high school, but Lisa had started getting involved in school activities that didn't interest Jenny, and Jenny's shyness also factored in. She really wasn't into sports, despite her physical education teacher saying she did well in them. She did, however, join the book club eventually, as she loved reading and writing stories.

She made three friends in Grade 9—Kayla Hennessy and two who were sisters Alyssa and Sarah Mailloux. Sarah had met Jenny through Alyssa as they were in the same grade. Sarah loved the fact that her sister had someone to talk to and share exciting news with, as Alyssa also had some issues to deal with. Sarah found her sister could be herself around Jenny and confide in her. Sarah remembers the sleepovers at our house and vice versa. They would all go to movies together or shopping and hockey games as well.

Sarah enjoyed tagging along when they went to the movies or Trick-or-Treating at Halloween, and they attended Jenny's birthday parties too. Kayla and Jenny had classes together and they also would have sleepovers at each other's places, and go together to each other's birthday parties, to the mall, and to movies. Jenny is still in contact with them all.

One girl whom Jenny thought was her friend and who spent time at our place, all of a sudden stopped talking to Jenny, or even acknowledging her existence. Jenny was very affected by this—she couldn't understand this girl's behaviour, as she hadn't done anything to warrant it, and this snubbing hurt her deeply. She thought she deserved an explanation, but never received one. Then another girl who knew this former friend of Jenny's did the same thing to her. This other girl bullied her too—they were so cruel. Jenny kept saying to me how she couldn't imagine ever treating anyone like that, especially without a reason.

Although it was still challenging for Jenny to converse, she tried harder and harder over time. She would become frustrated because she felt people didn't have the patience to wait for her to finish her thoughts or answer questions, and when she did manage to say something, it was as though they didn't consider it important or worth listening to. It didn't help that she wasn't "boy crazy" like many of them—she would tell me, "I have no time for boys as I want to do well in school and have my profession."

She was never really into serious fashion, either. I longed for the day she would dress a bit more "girly," and when she did occasionally wear a dress or a skirt she looked lovely. Of course, she looked great in her hoodies and jeans as well, but it was nice to see her try wearing something different. The important thing was she felt comfortable in her own skin, and I respected that. She wore her hair long and straight, and wasn't interested in my offers to style it. She would say to me "I am me and I don't have to be up on fashion or hairstyles. I like what I wear and how my hair is." She felt it was another reason why other girls and guys teased her and weren't interested in socializing with her. I was proud of her for not changing her style just to belong to a certain group—she was who she was.

Her language did advance, though her shyness and being quiet were what played on her. She was an introvert, not an extrovert; so it was hard for her to be overly sociable and outgoing at school. Jenny hated chatting on the phone and found it difficult to make conversation with friends and arrange to go out. So a lot of the time I would phone and schedule get-togethers on her behalf. She often felt she didn't say the right things, and it was awkward for her to try to keep conversations going.

There were two incidents that occurred during this time that were especially troubling to me. High school girls can of course be very mean, vindictive, and hurtful—both emotionally and physically. Once when Jenny was in the computer room working, a girl walked by and pushed her head forward so it hit the computer. When Jenny told me about it after school, I was ready to march right in there and track this girl down. But the way Jenny said, "Please leave it, Mum" told me she was scared of this girl. I explained to her that the girl's behaviour was not appropriate and should be dealt with, but I respected Jenny's wishes.

The second incident chills me to the bone every time I think of it. After the first incident, I had told Jenny to never be alone and to always make sure she was with one or more persons. On this day, she needed to get a report to one of her classes and thought it would only take a minute. As she was writing something on her paper, the girl from the first incident walked in, accompanied by a friend. She approached Jenny and started taunting her smugly, saying "Don't you want to be our friend? Come on, be our friend." Jenny asked the girl to please leave her alone so she could just submit her report. The girl gave her an evil look and left, only to return a minute later with a scarf in her hands. She wrapped the scarf around her own neck like a noose—to make it look like she was hanging herself—and said, "This is what you should do to yourself, because you're not worth living."

I was horrified and in shock when Jenny relayed this to me, and my whole being went numb. Jenny was so upset and I was livid. I got out of the van so fast and went straight to the counsellor and the principal. I wanted this girl found and her parents notified, as this was completely unacceptable. Fortunately, it was dealt with right away and this girl never bothered Jenny again. In my eyes, this went way beyond bullying—it boggles my mind how a young girl could treat another human being like that. At times, Jenny must have felt as though she was going into a war zone, trying to keep herself mentally and physically safe.

One thing we were trying to do both in and out of school was to get Jenny to be more assertive, as this was incredibly hard for her—she doesn't have an ill bone in her body, and she avoids conflict at all cost.

Jenny tried her best to not let it get her down when people looked at her funnily or made remarks about her. She was bound and determined to get through high school and graduate. No matter what she came up against—whether it was the bullying, studying, assignments, or the life of being a teenager—Jenny kept herself going, and I was always there for her. I constantly told her how much I believed in her, how smart she is, how beautiful she is inside and out, and how she deserves the best. I just kept telling her to trust me on that, which she always has.

When I was in the car and waiting to pick Jenny up from school or events, I would witness her shyness—no one talking to her and her being on her own. As a mother, all you pray for is that your child will be accepted and brought into the circle. I was happy though to see the change as high school went on.

Chapter Eleven

High School Years—The Second Half

Jenny went out of her regular classes from Grades 8 to 10 to do some subjects at the Learning Centre, which I'm sure the other kids noticed, and perhaps it cast a bit of a shadow over her. Jenny said it bothered her for kids to know; however, she knew that she had to do well in school and put up with what other kids said. Lisa Balcombe worked very hard with Jenny in the Learning Centre, and she and I would discuss where Jenny currently was, where she needed to be, and the best ways to support her progress.

When Jenny was fifteen years old and in Grade 10, Lisa administered a set of Woodcock-Johnson III Tests of Achievement. In her summary, Lisa said that Jenny's oral language skills were average when compared to the range of scores obtained by others her age, that her oral expression skills were low average, and that her listening comprehension skills were average. Compared to others at her age level, Jenny's academic skills, her ability to apply those skills, and her fluency with academic tasks were all within the low average range. Her level of academic knowledge and her performance in written expression was average; she achieved only low average in reading, basic reading skills, mathematics, math calculation, and basic writing skills. Areas of concern included math fluency, phonics, spelling of sounds, applied problem solving, and editing.

Her math teacher in Grades 9 and 10 commented to me on how organized she was and even though she had some struggles with math concepts, she faced them directly, readily accepted suggestions given to her, and learned from them. Jenny would always go the extra mile with her homework, saying, "I want to pass and get good marks, Mum."

Her math teacher said Jenny was always thorough with her assignments and well organized; that she was an independent student and that her work was outstanding. He was so thrilled to have her in both classes, and he told Jenny to be very proud of her efforts and achievements.

During Grade 10, Jenny really got into animation and would talk a great deal about it. As I thought about her love of animated movies and television shows, and how much she was enjoying art in school, I had a "lightbulb moment." I looked up "animation studios" in Vancouver online and came across Rainmaker Entertainment. I made an appointment in July 2009 with Justin Gladden, the Human Resource Manager at Rainmaker, and off we headed to Vancouver for Jenny to explore what animation entailed.

Justin was awesome and sensed how Jenny was drawn into animation. He gave us his business card and told me that I should start looking at animation schools and to contact him when she was finished high school. Jenny's eyes "bugged out" throughout the tour, and the smile on her face was the hugest I'd ever seen.

When we left she said to me "Mum, that was amazing and it is what I want to do. I really do." We were walking down one of the hallways when she stopped suddenly and said, "I wish I could be working here right now!" So, like everything else, I started my mission to get Jenny enrolled in an animation school.

It was around this time that Jenny got her first job. Julie, the manager at Taco Time® at Vernon Square Mall, was aware of Jenny's autism and special needs. One day she told me she needed an employee and asked Jenny if she would like to come on board. I knew Jenny was nervous and anxious when I looked at her. However, I felt this would be good for her and Julie was positive about having her work there. Jenny liked Julie, she trusted her and felt comfortable with her, and so she said she would give it a try.

Jenny loved working there, especially cooking and cleaning in the back, although she worked at the front as well. This meant looking after and talking with the customers, handling money at the till, making change, and processing debit and credit card charges. She expressed to me that she would rather be in the back cooking, as she said it made her anxious having to talk with people—she didn't want to say the wrong thing. She worried that she wouldn't understand them accurately.

Julie told me that Jenny was an excellent employee and very hard working. Her only area needing improvement was her speech level, and so Jenny tried her best to speak more loudly. This really was a breakthrough for Jenny as she never believed she would be able to handle such a responsibility.

Although she didn't know it, I would sometimes go to the mall to sit at a distance and watch her work. What a feeling it was for me to see her handling customers, making change, and cooking. I told her she should pat herself on the back, and what a huge accomplishment this was. I could tell she was feeling good about herself and enjoyed working there.

While it was hard at times serving people and taking care of orders, it helped her with conversation and handling money and, of course, she was making her own money as well! Jenny took great pride in that, and was amazing at saving her money. She would buy things she wanted; however, she was smart, and made sure she put money away for her future, as well. Sadly, Taco Time® closed down so her job came to an end. Even so, it was a blessing that she had had this opportunity. Jenny decided not to look for another job at this point, as she wanted to spend her time on schoolwork, her drawing, and writing.

By then, Jenny wasn't requiring the services of the Learning Centre as much, as she was doing so well on her own. She told me she didn't want to get help anymore—that she wanted to prove to herself that she could do this independently. I remember some of the teachers in the regular classes saying that Jenny had to be more open and ask questions if she didn't understand something in class. When I asked Jenny about this she said she would get nervous and worried she wouldn't ask the question correctly, and she didn't want to look dumb just because she didn't understand what was being taught. Jenny and I had many discussions about this, as it was imperative she ask questions; however, I recognized how hard it must have been for her.

So in Grades 11 and 12, Jenny did not go to the Learning Centre, but they let her know she could go there if she needed to. I honestly believe that the big changes launching the newfound belief in herself were her Grade 11 and 12 writing, art, clothing, and food classes, and the teachers who instructed them. These women really liked Jenny and believed in her, and this really brought her out of her shell. Her self-esteem received a huge boost when the teachers acknowledged her talent and communicated this to her. These experiences made coming to school for Jenny as relaxing as it could be in light of the other challenges she faced, knowing she could look forward to being in these classes.

Jenny loved her art classes. She enjoyed the challenge of each art piece and would go the extra mile. I remember some days coming into the school looking for her and finding her finishing her work in the art room. Even more so, she loved writing class, and she thought so much of her writing/English teacher, Mrs. Liz Wallberg. Jenny would tell me how Mrs. Wallberg liked a particular story she had written, and encouraged her to publish it, which surprised us both. Jenny's fellow students were also captivated with her story. As a matter a fact each student had been reading aloud a part of their stories each day, but everyone was so engaged in Jenny's story that they'd rather hear more of hers than their own so they could find out what was going to happen next.

Jenny's writing teacher, Mrs. Wallberg, believed in her hugely, and said that Jenny showed unfailing willingness to work, and gave her best effort in everything she did. She also told me that Jenny was a wonderful young writer and that she was crossing her fingers she would finish her book and get it published. She kept mentioning what a strong work ethic Jenny had, which was evidenced by the many "Worthy of Special Recognition" letters for outstanding work that both she and the school principal, Mr. Reed, awarded Jenny. I witnessed this at home as well, where Jenny put so much time and care into her homework for all subjects.

Another teacher who was impressed with Jenny was Mr. Gee, her Grades 11 and 12 history and social studies teacher. He commented that, in his experience, the number one ingredient for success is a willingness to stick with the challenge and keep chipping away at it, and he thanked Jenny for modelling this to the other students. He told Jenny and me at our parent interview with him that, in her final exam, Jenny was in the top eight of her class, which showed her commitment to learning the material. We went out and celebrated that day after hearing such news!

One teacher who put a smile on my face was Jenny's fine arts and drama teacher, Ms. Collinson. She told me Jenny was attentive, on time, and enthusiastic, and that in time she improved substantially in her level of confidence on stage. She did say though that her voice was still quiet, but that her physical character was coming through, loud and strong. Why this affects me is that Jenny would come home and tell me that she didn't like going on stage and acting in front of people. She said it made her uncomfortable and wasn't for her. She says to this day she likes being behind the scenes and not in front, like with her animation. Anyhow, I was proud that she persisted with it, even though it made her anxious.

Others teachers would commend her work ethic as well and her positive attitude, her smile, and her patience, and how conscientious she was—many of them said her future looked so bright. One teacher said she would bet Jenny was one of the hardest working students in the school and she couldn't say enough good things about her. Her art teacher, Mrs. De Langen, told me that Jenny's talent and passion were very evident in her work, and that she was so happy to have Jenny for all three years of art. I was truly blown away when she would bring her artwork home—talented—yes, but most of all it was to see Jenny's joy when she drew.

Her fellow students wrote in Jenny's Grade 11 Yearbook that she had such a great imagination she should never stop writing. These great compliments from her peers really brought Jenny out, and helped with her self-esteem. I spoke to a couple of students one day outside the English classroom, and they told me how much they enjoyed Jenny's book and praised her talent. Jenny just smiled and was her humble self once more; however, I knew it gave her such a good feeling and a sense of belonging—of being liked. It truly was a turning point for her, both personally and professionally, and I was ecstatic for her.

Jenny was now interested in both animation and writing. I remember her at home spending many hours writing her book and drawing illustrations of her characters. Papers and pencils were everywhere. She was so absorbed in it and loved me to read the chapters as she wrote them, and to look at the pictures. It was a very engaging story with characters that drew me in—I couldn't wait to read the next page! Jenny was finally happy with where she was in her life and what she wanted to do.

She kept up her art classes right through Grade 12 and

continued to receive great marks. It was the same with her writing and English classes where chapters of her book constantly entertained her teacher and fellow writing students. She could see her future starting to surface and become a reality. Jenny worked tirelessly in all her subjects and received many certificates for awards and achievements throughout her years at Fulton. She achieved marks way higher than expected. She was chipping off her autism challenges bit by bit and accomplishing academic miracles.

Jenny's progress prompted me to reach out to Vancouver Film School, which I had heard had one of the best animation programs, not only in North America, but in the world. They had people from every country wanting to get into their school. I made an appointment for Jenny on Friday, April 30, 2010 with the Admissions Officer, Scott Williams.

The day of the appointment, off Jenny and I went to Vancouver to meet up with Scott and learn all about VFS's animation courses. I remember Jenny looking at me and saying, "Oh, Mum, I will never get in here."

I said, "Trust me, Jenny, I know you will! All your hard work, plus our determination as a mother-and-daughter team ... all your dreams will come true."

We had a super meeting with Scott. He was a lovely fellow and really liked Jenny and her story. He gave me all the information of what was needed to apply for the courses as Jenny wanted to do both 2D Classical Animation and 3D Digital Character Animation.

It was unbelievable what VFS expected to be handed in for the application. Jenny said, "There is no way—I don't think my drawing is good enough and so many people will be applying."

I looked at her and said, "You are just as good an artist as anyone else, and your hard work ethic, attitude, and passion for animation will see you through. I believe in you and you must trust me." I also told her to look back over her life so far, and to acknowledge how far she had come— all she had achieved and conquered when I had been told she'd never be able to. So I said to her, "Nothing can stop you from doing this either. You can achieve this as well; it is in you." I told her to trust herself, to respect herself, and love herself as she was a special, unique human being and this was her calling in this world: to be an animator, a storyteller.

She looked at me and said, "Thanks, Mum, for believing in me and always being here for me. I love you."

So the next couple of years in high school, she worked extremely hard, which was reflected both in her marks as well as in the comments from all her teachers. She received a multitude of A grades and was in the Graduation Program with Honours. This was so impressive considering where her life had begun and the limitations she had faced and in some instances continued to face. She has had ups and downs with peers and socialization, and she has had to push tirelessly through with certain subjects, but she did it with her cheering squad by her side: me, Chris, Travis, and last but not least her dog, Mr. Sparkles.

We contacted Scott Williams at VFS again when Jenny was just starting Grade 12, and let him know Jenny wanted to apply for 2D Classical and 3D Digital Character Animation Classes. He was so happy to hear this and got everything started for her to apply. There was a lot that had to be done with the application. Her school marks would be considered, of course, and we would need references from teachers (Mrs. Wallberg and Mr. Gee gladly obliged). Lin Oldfield, her Respite Care worker, did one as well. The Board of the Vancouver Film School was very taken by her references.

What Others Shared: Mrs. Wallberg's Reference Letter to VFS

"I am very pleased to be asked to write a letter of reference for Jenny Story. Jenny has been a student in my school and in my classroom. She has participated in two of the writing classes our school offers. During Jenny's time with me I was struck with her commitment to her writing. She worked tirelessly on a novel for pre-teens. Her delightful sense of humour was evident in her work. She showed a wonderful willingness to critique other writers' work. Her openness to others and her quiet confidence added immensely to my classes. She would be a wonderful asset to any school program she joins. She has struggled through some amazing challenges and kept that wondrous positivity in everything she does."

What Others Shared: Lin Oldfield's Reference Letter to VFS

"I am and have been Jenny Story's Respite Care Worker for the past fifteen years, since she was three years old. It has been my pleasure to spend time with her and it has been a delight to see the changes in her during that time. Those changes have been huge. She has worked diligently to get herself to the place she is at now. Because of her autism, she has struggled in social situations, but through her hard work and determination she is overcoming the challenges that autism brings. She has always had a love of art. She works conscientiously, paying great attention to detail, constantly trying to improve her abilities, and learn from others, from books, and the internet. She is a very well-mannered, honest, caring young lady. It has been my pleasure to have been Jenny's respite care worker."

Jenny had to provide them with a lot of art work. I remember one form was Body Art—she had some from art class and they were fantastic. I even modelled for some of her pieces of art as well, which was quite the learning experience for me, both watching her work and being her model. There was also a lot of paperwork regarding admission, finances, grants, scholarships, and much more that I had to deal with and fill out; however it was all worth it. It took up a lot of time and there was a deadline. I give Jenny credit as she was in her last year of school and was under a lot of pressure with schoolwork and wanting to graduate. She worked exceptionally hard in both areas, and finished all the art work that needed to be done before the animation school deadline, then sent everything off to VFS.

Then the waiting game began.

Jenny was so busy with her schooling that it kept her mind off her VFS application somewhat. I was thinking positively, and I knew and felt she would get in. My heart still skipped a beat the day I opened the mailbox and saw the envelope, however. Jenny had told me she wanted me to open it when the mail arrived, as she wouldn't be able to as she was anxious about what it might say. Plus, it came when she was at school.

I unfolded the letter and began to read.

"Dear Jenny, this letter is to verify that you meet the entrance requirements and have been accepted into the 2011-08-29 to 2012-08-17 year of Classical Animation. You will be required to attend a student wide orientation, which will take place on 2011-08-22. It is imperative that you initial, sign and return the enclosed Enrollment Form. On behalf of the Administration and Faculty of VFS, congratulations on your acceptance."

I was screaming so loudly and jumping so high, the neighbours must have thought something was wrong. It was the happiest day of my life—for her—and to think I had been told not to expect much! How Jenny had turned that around.

I drove right away to the store and bought a bouquet of balloons, streamers, and a helium balloon with "Congratulations" on it. I placed the acceptance papers in a card and I went to the office at Fulton to ask if I could go and see Jenny in her classroom. The receptionists knew Jenny and me, and were so happy for her that they said no problem and to go for it. They gave me the classroom number to her video editing class.

I was running down the hallways to find the room. When I found it, I stopped to catch my breath and noticed the classroom was dark, as they were watching something. I knocked on the door and her teacher said, "Come in," and there were all the students and the teacher looking at me, wondering what was going on. I told the teacher this would just take a minute. I raced up to Jenny and gave her a big hug and kiss and then gave her the balloon bouquet and card, and shouted excitedly to her, "You got in; you have been accepted for the Animation Program at Vancouver Film School."

Initially, she was just stunned that I was in her classroom, but then it slowly hit her that her dream was coming true. Her eyes popped wide open and people began congratulating her. I thanked her teacher for letting me do this, and he said, "No problem," and congratulated Jenny as well.

I took Jenny out for supper at Kelly O'Bryan's, one of her favourite restaurants, to celebrate her acceptance. Jenny said to me that when I left the classroom she was so happy, but was also asking herself what had just happened.

Scott told me that the VFS Board was very excited to have Jenny at the school and welcomed her with open arms. Jenny and I danced, cried, jumped up and down, and could now breathe comfortably: she was going to animation school! I knew it, I believed in her and most of all, this young lady richly deserved it.

Amidst the celebration, we did realize that there was still a lot of work that had to be done. First she needed to finish Grade 12 and graduate. We had to get her all ready for Grad, so first we had to buy a dress, shoes, and jewellery—which was going to be exciting and fun to do. I couldn't wait to see my daughter in a full-length gown with her hair done up and make-up on. Jenny told me she could see how excited I was and joked about me getting to see her in a dress. She said to me, "Hey, Mum, a dream of yours is coming true too." We both had a good laugh about that.

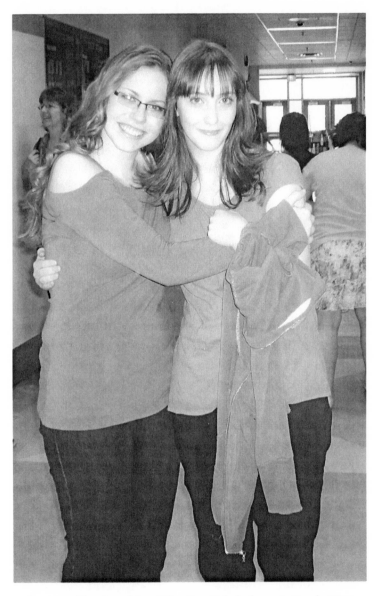

Jenny and her best friend Lisa Rae-Babchuk are in Grade 12 at Clarence Fulton High School.

What Others Shared: Lisa Rae-Babchuk

I spoke to Lisa recently and she told me of her memories and friendship with Jenny.

"Jenny is smart and independent in ways that make her successful now. In High School we were not in a lot of the same classes, maybe six classes together in those five years. Any time Jenny needed help, she never asked for the answer. The teacher or I could re-explain the question or expand on what it wanted for an answer, but Jenny always wanted her own answer. She would get to the point, 'Oh, I get it,' and start writing like crazy. She never copied other people's work or tried to take the easy way out. She worked hard for her marks and always tried her best. That is how she made it to this point today. She just kept working at what she loves."

What Others Shared: Cierra Carlyle

"Jenny is a very talented young lady as well and she bonded with people over art and creative writing. I always loved looking at her original drawings and comics. They were always so cute and quirky. I remember one day sitting in our Grade 12 Video/ Computer class and Jenny's Mum came into the room saying, 'Jenny, you got into animation school.'

"I gave her a big hug because I knew at that moment all her hard work and struggles had been worth it. It was crazy to think of Jenny going off to the big city of Vancouver to go after her dream, but I knew it was the best possible thing for her to do.

We both went right into intense programs but that didn't stop our friendship. We mostly connect in emails, but I sometimes get the chance to go visit her in Vancouver, and it's amazing to be with my best friend again. I was so unbelievably proud of her when she told me she got a deal to publish a book. It shows that if you work hard enough, no matter what the circumstances, you can achieve your dreams. She has come so far since that Grade 8 English class and I can't wait to see where she goes and I will be there to support her every step of the way."

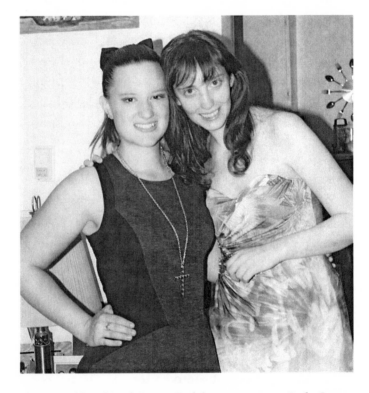

Jenny and her friend Cierra Carlyle prepare to see Lady Gaga.

Chapter Twelve

A Fundraiser, Graduation, and Other Events

In Jenny's last year of high school, I promoted and planned a fundraising dance and silent auction to help cover costs for the animation schooling. It would be very expensive and she was planning to do two separate programs covering two years of schooling. The scholarships were great and she did get some grants; however, we needed as much help as we could get.

My friend Jackson Mace has a band called "Maceland" that was on board to play for the fundraising dance—he knew the lady at Elks Hall and she gave us the hall rental for free. I had never met this woman before and when she heard Jenny's story she let us have the hall. What a beautiful, kind lady she was. I had the tickets and posters printed, and did a lot of marketing and promoting for the event. The poster had a lovely picture of Jenny on it with a photo of Jackson's band and the heading, "Jenny Story's Road to Animation Fundraising Dance." We posted them all over the city and sold tickets from a local eatery as well. Plus, we had a silent auction, for which a lot of local businesses donated lovely items. My friend Maureen Ruscheinsky was a blessing, as she was the leader of the silent auction.

I spoke with Brian Martin at Sun FM Radio Station and explained what I was doing, and he was very receptive to having us on his morning *Sunrise Show*. So was Betty Selin, his morning show counterpart. Brian made the interview so comfortable and informative about Jenny and the dance. We had a lot of fun.

Brian helped Jenny out as she was extremely nervous. She had said to me prior, "Mum, I don't think I can do this. What if I can't get the questions right?" I told her that I would be right beside her to help if she didn't understand a question. We talked about Jenny's history, her journey, and the purpose of the fundraiser for her film school fees. We were very grateful to Brian, Betty, and the radio station for letting us come on.

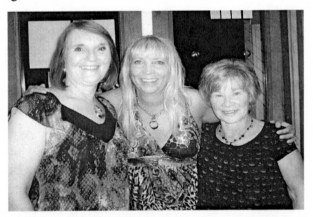

I am with my two favourite Respite Care Givers and friends, Lin Oldfield and Lucy McInnes, at Jenny's Fundraising Dance.

The dance was a lot of work but so worthwhile. Jenny said she saw the love for her and for our family in Vernon. When the day of the event arrived, we were up early getting the hall decorated with streamers, balloons, and big poster pictures of Jenny. One was her graduation picture, another from when she was little, and the last one was as a teenager. They lit up the room and showed the essence of Jenny.

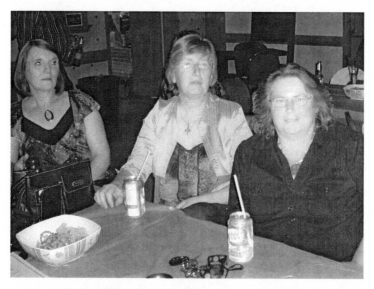

Left to right, Lin Oldfield, Deb Radies, and Gail Cunningham attend Jenny's fundraising dance. Deb and Gail own Brer Rabbit Day Care.

There was hot food, snacks, and drinks. We also had a 50/50 Draw. It was a fun evening and you could see everyone enjoying themselves. It was heart-warming to see all of Jenny's Dream Team, the staff from Brer Rabbit Day Care, and our Respite Care Workers. We had great talks with them all night, and Jenny and I presented them with gifts, flowers, and cards later in the evening to personally thank each of them for everything they had done for us.

These people have played a huge part in bringing Jenny to where she is. We did the same for everyone who helped us with the dance, as we were so grateful for their help and support. To see Jenny having so much fun with her friends that evening, dancing up a storm, was invaluable.

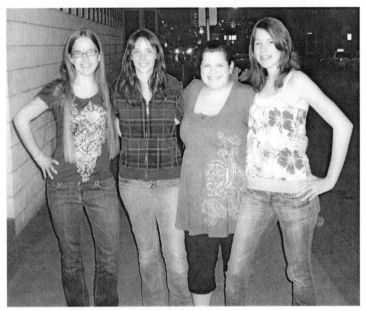

Alyssa, Jenny, Kayla, and Sarah pose for the camera at Jenny's fundraising dance

What Others Shared: Guest Book Comments

We had a guest book, and received so many lovely comments.

Gail Cunningham and Deb Radies from Brer Rabbit wrote: "Go, Girl, Go. We always knew you would fly and so you are. We are so proud of you and all you have accomplished through all your hard work and your determination. We know you will continue to soar."

From Lin Oldfield: "You are one amazing young lady. It has been such a privilege to have been part of your life for fifteen years. You have grown and matured in so many ways. I'm so proud of you. I'm going to miss you more than words can say. Love ya!"

From Bob Oldfield (Lin's husband): "What an exciting time awaits you. Lin and I are so excited for you and look forward to hearing all the reports of how you're doing. It's been great to have you as part of our family all these years. We'll really miss you. Have the greatest time. Best wishes and lots of love."

From Darlene Wolsey: "Jenny, I am so happy for you. You have made some amazing accomplishments! I have enjoyed my opportunity to be a small part of your life and to know your family. Your mom is a fantastic lady. All the very best to you in all that you do. You Go Girl!"

From Margaret Hudson: "Dear Jenny, I am so glad for you-I wish you all the best in Vancouver. You are amazing. You deserve to have all your dreams come true. It has been a pleasure helping you and your family, and a privilege to be part of your journey. Blessings. And to you, Janet and Travis, what wonderful parents you are. You must be very proud of Jenny, love and best wishes."

From Ann Cordingly: "I still always think of how beautiful and serene you looked one night at a Powerhouse party. I know you will excel at the animation course. You are so lucky to have such support from your family."

From Kayla Hennessy: "Jenny, I am so happy and proud of you, sweetie. You worked so hard to get where you are. I am so happy that you get to live your dream. I am going to miss you so much. You deserve this as you are an amazing artist, and you are amazing and sweet. Your dream has come true, live it up, and soak up every minute. You rock, can't wait to Grad with you."

These comments really meant a lot to us and showed Jenny once more who she is and how much her friends all love her.

I experienced so many emotions when Jenny's High School Graduation day arrived—happiness, pride, joy, and my engulfing love for my daughter. However, at the same time it was hard to see her all grown up and not our little girl anymore. As I watched her try on grad dresses, I was flooded with memories of her life leading up to this point. It was priceless to see her coming out in different dresses and looking at herself in the mirror, as I thought back to when she was a little girl and did not even look in a mirror, or talk or socialize. And now here she was trying on beautiful dresses and discussing them with the saleswoman. She was all grown up and looked like a princess.

She had her own ideas and opinions on the dresses, of course. Time stood still when she came out in a white and silver-flecked strapless gown and my jaw dropped. She looked like a model. I do not think Jenny realizes how gorgeous she looked; how elegantly she wore the gown. I did see her smile grow bigger and a gleam come in her eyes, and we looked at one another and knew this one was the winner—we bought it there and then. We had hair and make-up appointments all set up. Next on our agenda was to get shoes and jewellery. We found the perfect silver, sparkly, stone-coloured shoes that matched with the dress like they were born together. We came across a lovely drop necklace and a bracelet to match, and the sweetest ring in the shape of a bow. She wore my mother's earrings as well, which warmed my heart. Jenny didn't want pierced ears, and these clip-on ones went beautifully with her dress. My mum had passed away in 2001—she would have been so proud of Jenny's progress, especially since she was with me at the testing and evaluation early on, and had seen first-hand how Jenny used to be. She would be so happy for Jenny and all her accomplishments and who she had become.

Deb and Gail from Brer Rabbit Day Care surprised Jenny when they came by the house to give her a graduation present. Jenny could not believe her eyes as it was a high-tech Canon camera. They knew Jenny loved photography and was good at it. These two have always been so thoughtful to Jenny, so generous.

When the morning of graduation day arrived, I remember Jenny looking at me and saying, "Mum, I can't believe it. I passed Grade 12 and got accepted to Vancouver Film School."

I replied, "Of course you did. I've always believed in you."

That morning she had her hair and make-up done. She had never worn make-up before—she said she only wore lip gloss so her lips wouldn't chap. Jenny's good friend Lisa was there getting her make-up done as well, and they were all excited, talking, and giggling.

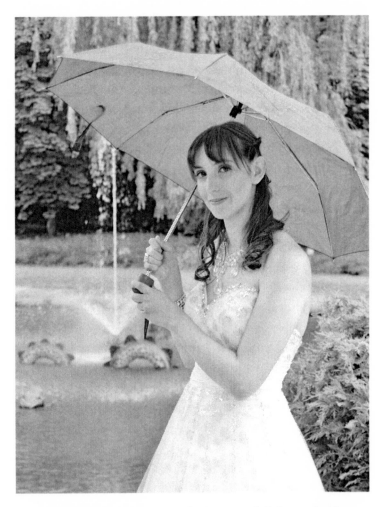

This is my favourite picture of Jenny out of all the graduation photos we had taken at Polson Park in Vernon.

When the time came to put on the dress and ensemble, Jenny took our breath away—she looked stunning. She was all grown up. We headed off to her Graduation Ceremony where she had to get into her cap and gown. It was a lovely ceremony and when Jenny walked across to receive her Graduation Certificate, we were cheering our heads off and streaming with happy tears. My sister Vicki came out for it, as did our friends Gail and Deb from Brer Rabbit—Gail's niece was graduating as well and other friends, one being my good friend, Terry O'Sullivan. Jenny had done it! All her hard work and challenges, trooping through the barricades, she graduated, she passed Grade 12! Everything she had gone through could be thrown out the window. She had proved to herself that she had reached her goal and showed everyone else she could do it and then some.

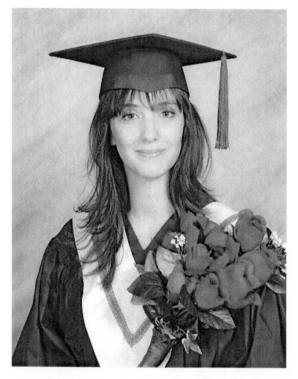

Jenny smiles in her cap and gown at her Grade 12 Graduation.

When she accepted her Grade 12 Certificate, she was held on stage as she was about to be given a scholarship. Her face was priceless—talk about a wonderful surprise. We all screamed out her name and were jumping up and down. She received the 2011 Silver Star Rotary Club Achievement Award, in addition to a scholarship she had already received from the Powerhouse Theatre. We also found out that Jenny was selected to receive the $500 Passport of Education Award for Grade 12, which recognizes a student's achievement in a range of academic and non-academic areas.

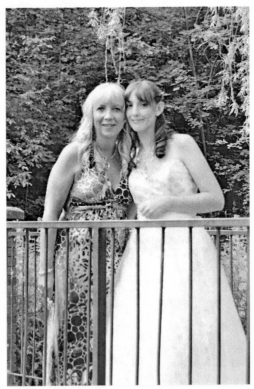

Mother and daughter enjoy a special day together, a dream come true.

Time stood still for me at this moment as I considered everything she and I had gone through from her birth right up to this ceremony. Watching Jenny graduate from high school, receive scholarships, be accepted to Vancouver Film School for animation, and seeing her evolve into this beautiful, classy, intelligent, and talented young lady were thrills beyond words.

To think how bleak and dim her future had been foreseen by some and to see her now, I know dreams do come true; the light does glow at the end of the dark tunnel. My daughter Jenny is a prime example and role model for this.

As parents we need to provide the future our children deserve—grow with them, learn from them, strive for them, fight for them, and believe in them. We need to help them reach for their rainbow, their pot of gold, and let their dreams soar. Jenny so deserved this, and I was elated to see her absorbing this and believing in herself.

I was on the parental board for the after party for the students and we had organized a dance for them. It was a lovely sight to see Jenny dancing with Travis, and it was hard for him not to shed tears. She kept saying, "It's okay, Dad, come on."

Also we had a big carnival set up with games and events for them to do, which Travis and I worked at as well. We could see Jenny was having so much fun and participating in it all. She won the jousting challenge against her opponent, as she is a strong girl. At times, she would look over at us and give us that beautiful smile of hers.

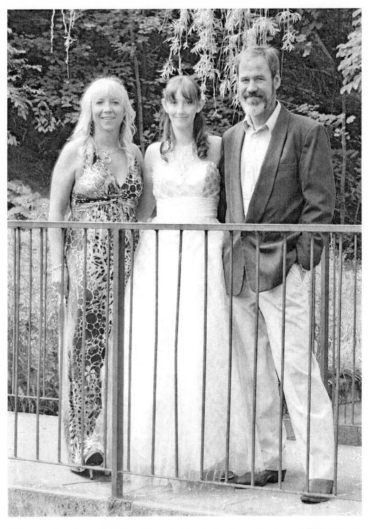

The graduation photographer takes one of me, Jenny, and Travis at
Polson Park.

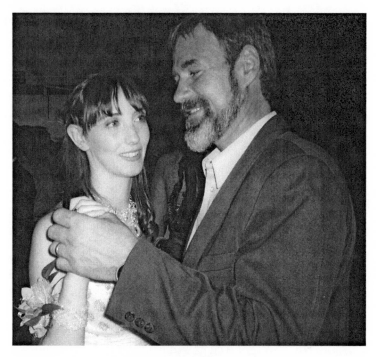

Jenny and Travis dance at her graduation at Clarence Fulton High School.

What Others Shared: Lucy McInnes

"As she got older [Jenny] would talk to me about some of her issues at school and with friends and socialization. We also would go out to the movies. There were two movies that we saw and especially liked: *Ice Age* and *Polar Bear Express*.

"She was always upfront and honest. I remember her writing her book and telling me about it and I even read a couple of chapters. I really enjoyed it; it was so well done. I have many a fond memory of Jenny and I am so happy for her and so proud of her for all that she has accomplished. In seeing all she went through and where she is now, I know she is a role model. It was a pleasure and joy to be at her Fundraising Dance her Mum put on for her. Janet and I became good friends and had many good chats and laughs. I feel honoured to be a part of her journey and in getting to know her and Janet and Travis. I wish Jenny continuing success and happiness."

Something exciting came out of our interview on Sun FM Radio. A woman named Wendy Battersby heard it on her car radio and started crying. She went and told her husband, Darren Battersby, and then she called the radio station and wanted Brian to give her our phone number as they wanted to meet and talk to us about something. Her husband wanted to help Jenny and give her an opportunity for her animation classes.

We arranged to meet them at a Red Robin® restaurant. They were so nice and, to our surprise, her husband was an employee of Bardel Entertainment Inc.'s animation studios in Vancouver. He told us that he had talked to the owners of Bardel—Barry Ward and his wife Delna Bhesania—who wanted to meet Jenny and invited us to brunch in Kelowna. Jenny and I were pinching ourselves—who would have thought this young girl from Vernon, after everything she had gone through, would already be meeting the owners of the well-known Bardel Animation Studio. They work with DreamWorks Studios, Fox, Nickelodeon, and more!

We drove to Kelowna and Jenny brought her art and storyboard work. We met them at the Grand Hotel and had a wonderful conversation over our meal while they looked at her art work. Suddenly, a man came to join us, and we discovered he was the Head of Production in Los Angeles for Nickelodeon, Dean Huff. Jenny was stunned and on cloud nine. She had a really great talk with him as he looked at all her work. Dean gave her great compliments and loved her storyboards. He also gave her his personal business card and said to call him and to come down anytime and he would take her on a tour through Nickelodeon Studios. I was as proud as punch watching her talk about her work with these people.

On our drive home, Jenny was beyond excited. She said, "Mum, he liked my story boards, he gave me his card and said to go down there." Such a cherished memory for Jenny to hold, as well as a nice lead up for her heading into animation school.

We were both very grateful to Barry and his wife for wanting to meet us in Kelowna—it was so lovely of them. We have since got together with Barry a couple of times, toured through his animation studio, and also been out for lunch with him—and met a young gal and guy he knew from the States who had autism and who worked in the animation field. It was such a joy to meet and talk with them and their families. We couldn't believe all of this transpired simply from talking about a fundraising dance on the radio—who would have thought that the wife of a Bardel employee would be listening to the radio at that time?

Our excitement didn't end there, as in February we went to the local newspaper, the *Vernon Morning Star* and met up with Editor Katherine Mortimer, who wrote a full-page article on Jenny and her story. It was called, "Jenny takes an 'Animated Journey'" and the subtitle was, "A love of drawing will take Jenny Story on a journey from High School Graduation to the animation program at the Vancouver Film School." We have the article hanging up on the living room wall as a reminder for Jenny. There was a picture of her in the middle of the article with a caption that read, "Grade 12 Student Jenny Story works on a drawing in the art room at Fulton Secondary School."

The opening paragraph said, "Thanks to a mother's love and a daughter's determination, the future is filled with possibilities for Jenny Story. And as she walks up on stage to collect her High School Diploma in June, it will be the end of one chapter and the beginning of another. The 17-year-old Honours Student will leave Vernon this summer and begin her studies at Vancouver Film School. It has been a long journey and would seem impossible at the beginning. But Janet Walmsley was determined that her daughter's future would be as bright as any other youngster's."

The article went on to talk about Jenny's visit to Vancouver, the specialists, tests, and the bleak outlook. It also talked about her getting very ill after her inoculations and how she changed to a whole different child, as well as the people who banded together to help her. The article then went on to mention her socialization challenges and my concerns for her.

In her interview, Jenny said, "I always liked to do art because it comforted me. High school was scary because I had trouble talking to people. But with certain teachers and certain classes, I had fun, especially with Mrs. Wallberg, Mr. Gee, and Mrs. Harrison, who all really believed in me and I am where I am because of them." The article described my praise for all who worked with Jenny, and especially her brother Chris and her dad, Travis. It also described the struggles and challenges she faced in high school.

The article highlighted her love of animation and animated movies and how she was a natural fit for Vancouver Film School. Jenny said to Katherine, "I was really excited at first and still am; however, now I am also nervous because this is a new experience, but it is one worth taking and I'm glad my mom is going with me." It went on to say how we were looking forward to exploring more of Vancouver and how I will be pursuing my acting career, continuing the work for which I was familiar to Vernon audiences through the Powerhouse Theatre.

I responded, "We're both following our dreams."

The article also touched on how a counsellor had told me that Jenny is a miracle—for a child to do what she has accomplished—from where she was at three years old, through kindergarten, to now—is so rare it's almost unbelievable. Katherine also kindly mentioned at the end that we had an account set up for Jenny at the local Credit Union if there were local businesses or individuals who wished to contribute for Jenny to pursue her dream.

Katherine ended the article with me saying, "Their

donation or scholarship would be in the good hands of a girl who is so hard working, smart, honest, respectful, and kind, and who deserves to see her dreams come true. We're hoping people can help her and be a part of her dream." It really was an eye-opening article about Jenny and we appreciated Katherine doing this for us.

After Jenny finished high school and was getting ready to move to Vancouver, I received a letter from the school principal at Fulton, Mr. Malcolm Reid. He said, "I am pleased to inform you that Jenny has been named to the Grade 12 Honour Roll of Distinction for the 2010/2011 year. To achieve this a student must earn an A- 86% average and a full course load. We felt this achievement of Jenny's was worthy of special recognition and I join with the teachers in offering congratulations to Jenny and to keep up the good work and study habit." This was a lovely way for Jenny to end high school.

There was a lot of paperwork to be done for animation schooling in connection with finances and grants, etc. Plus there was a lot of paperwork involved in applying for the Social Assistance for which Jenny qualified. We found out in April that her application was approved. The authorities said Jenny was eligible for grant funding through the Canada Student Grant for Persons with Permanent Disabilities for all years of post-secondary study.

Jenny received grants through Permanent Disability of BC and Canada, and also received a BC Student Loan and a Canada Student Loan. Travis and I had to put our own personal money toward the courses as well. I was working a full-time job and with all this happening we needed to find a place in Vancouver to move to. Travis and I were selling our home and going with Jenny. Our friend Maureen Ruscheinsky was our realtor.

There was so much to prepare to make sure the place always looked presentable for showings. Jenny's schooling started in late August, so we had to act fast to find a home in Vancouver, as we had only found out in February that she was accepted. Jenny and I travelled there on the weekends and spent hours looking at apartments. We covered a lot of territory and finally hit the jackpot and found a place that had everything we wanted, in addition to taking pets; Mr. Sparkles was family and we had to make sure he could be with us.

We found the place in June and rented it for mid-July as we wanted to have at least a month to get moved in, settled, and familiar with where her school was. Travis's job had him out of town a lot, so I had to take care of all this. In the meantime, Maureen was successful at selling our home, though, we took a loss as we needed to sell quickly.

The move was sad as we had lived in Vernon for seventeen years and we loved it there. Jenny at this point could not live on her own and we had no family or friends in Vancouver, so I wasn't letting her go alone. She deserved this opportunity and I wanted to do everything I could to be there for her and make her as comfortable as possible. When you have gone through this journey and seen all that your child has gone through, how she battled all the odds and worked extremely hard, selling the house and moving was no big deal. And that is what I did—gave her the world, to follow her dreams and achieve them. Jenny has always said how thankful and grateful she is to us and for being here with her as it means a lot to her.

Postscript: Mercedes Fraser

On August 17, 2012, a tragedy happened that hit us hard. I received a phone call from Sharlene Fraser, Mercedes' mum. I mentioned in an earlier chapter that Mercedes and Jenny were buddies for many years when they were little. When Jenny left for high school, they had different friends and drifted apart. However, when Mercedes started going to Fulton we gave her rides to school and we would catch up on what she was up to.

It was with heavy hearts that we found out that Mercedes had been killed. It was a tragic and senseless death as she was hit by a car when riding her bike to work. She was not at fault as the woman driver fell asleep at the wheel and ran over her. Mercedes was only seventeen years old and had such a bright future ahead of her. She would have been graduating Grade 12; she was going to be accepted as a nominee for Silver Star Queen in Vernon; and she had mapped out so much more for her life.

Jenny and I cherish all the memories and times we had with Mercedes.

What Others Shared: Lisa Rae-Babchuk, Later

"I love Jenny's mature thinking. It's the same thinking she's always had. She thinks about things in the long-term and how they will impact her whole life. It's what makes her work hard, like being brave enough to write a book and send it off to get published and apply for animation school and complete it. Jenny doesn't have to make a goal to accomplish anything, she just decides to do it and does it. I did worry about how Jenny would do in a different city and how would it be for her to make friends. But Jenny is such a spectacular person I didn't have to worry, but I still do as I want the best for her."

Jenny and I went to Lisa's wedding in November 2013. Lisa was so happy to have Jenny there, being so supportive and showing that she could see how much Lisa loved Clinton.

Lisa said "Jenny is the best friend in the whole world as she is honest and doesn't judge. When something good happens to someone she is genuinely happy for them and doesn't get jealous. She is sweet and kind and Jenny is one of the best people on this planet and I am so grateful to have her as my friend."

Chapter Thirteen

Vancouver and Animation School

Our new adventure was about to begin. We finished cleaning up the house after our belongings had been packed into the moving van. Our vehicle was so crammed there wasn't even room to breathe inside. Mr. Sparkles was cramped but he was a trooper the whole drive to Vancouver, and Jenny ensured he was as comfortable as possible and had many extra treats. We had acquired a lot in the seventeen years we had lived in Vernon, and ended up getting rid of three truckloads worth of stuff. We were downsizing from a three-bedroom home with a big shed to a much smaller two-bedroom apartment.

Jenny was excited about our new home, as it had a dishwasher, and a separate bathroom she could call her own; but I had mixed feelings as we said our final goodbyes to our neighbours, our home, and Okanagan Lake. Jenny said goodbye to her friends as well and told me it would be hard not to hang out with them, but she was happy to be leaving and going to Vancouver. I did not see any routine change issues with her on this move. I saw a young woman excited about where her life was going—she was happy and looking forward to what lay ahead.

I had made many long-time friends, too; the Okanagan is a slice of heaven. I would miss the people at Powerhouse Theatre, where I acted in a lot of plays—even directing a show and being on the Board. I had also been doing films in Kelowna for the Okanagan Society of Independent Filmmakers and at the Centre for Arts and Technology, Okanagan. I was fortunate, however, that I could work my actual job from home, so it could move anywhere with me. However, I must say for myself in going to Vancouver, it was a bonus for my acting career. Travis was working out of town on the day we headed to Vancouver, so we were on our own driving and setting up. We drove out of the carport slowly as Jenny and I looked at each other and slapped a high five. I said, "Our journey has now begun" as we both smiled with excitement. We took a deep breath and never looked back.

Once we were settled into our new home, Jenny and I starting exploring Vancouver and seeing what was close by in our area. Jenny was thrilled to discover there is a Tim Hortons® close by, so life was good for her. We are in an area where we are close to a lot of things and a short drive to her school. Bus and skytrain are close by too. It is a fabulous spot. We are also near Granville Island and can walk down to the ocean, and there is a huge dog park with a waterfall pond area for Sparkles.

I was really happy to see how much Jenny loves it here, and that Vancouver feels like home to her. I like it myself as well, as there is so much to do and see. People are so friendly and nice. Travis was not so keen on Vancouver, it being a big city. He is a small-town guy and likes the bush, so it was a bit of an adjustment for him. He recognized though that this is what Jenny deserves and needs, so he fully understands. As an ironworker, he has to be out of town a lot, and he misses his "girls," as he says. My hubby and daughter hugged me and said I did a great job finding a place in a good area—I felt so, too!

Before VFS's orientation and starting class, I thought it would be a good idea for Jenny to have a look at the school and classrooms so she would have a good feel for the environment and the teachers. Dieter, who was head of Senior Classical Animation, said he would love to meet and talk with Jenny. The administrator Vanessa said she would love to meet Jenny too and show her all around so she would be familiar with her new school. We met them in early August at the campus on Burrard Street, which was less than a ten-minute drive from where we live. We had a great meeting with Dieter and Vanessa as they talked about the school and the classes, after which they asked Jenny if she had any questions. Then Vanessa took us all around and showed Jenny the classrooms she would be in, the cafeteria, computer rooms, and washrooms. Jenny was glowing and I could see she couldn't wait to start. We were very grateful to Dieter and Vanessa for meeting up with us and making Jenny's first day a lot easier.

On that same day of meeting Dieter and Vanessa, we went to see Scott, the Admissions Advisor at VFS, whom we had met at the very beginning. He was at the other campus on West Hastings, and there we discussed the next program Jenny wanted to take, 3D Digital Character Animation. We got things rolling for this next course so she could go right into it after finishing the 2D Classical Animation Program. Scott was very informative and organized, making the application for Jenny to enter animation school smooth sailing. Shannon Brett was an assistant in the administration area and she helped me out a lot with the financial aspect and grants.

Jenny's Orientation Day was on August 27, 2011, and was held at the Scotiabank Theatre on Burrard. The orientation was for all courses; it was a packed house. Parents and one guest were invited to come, and I was happy to be a part of this with Jenny. It was well-organized and they showed an informative film introducing the school, staff, and graduates of the school. They had everyone yell out for each course they were in. Jenny got to know and meet a few people. We were there the whole morning and then the next day, it was—boom—right into classes. No wasting time, that is for sure. This course ran right from August 27, 2011 straight through to August 17, 2012. There were no breaks, no summer holidays; it was continuous.

Students were given all the outlines of information about the six courses to be covered throughout the whole year in 2D Classical Animation. There were also additional non-credit sessions that a student could take. Jenny took those as well and loved them as she wanted to engulf herself in everything. A photo was taken for their pass card to be able to get in and out of the building. Security was really high; it was hard to get in if they forgot their building access card. For a parent, it was good to see the great security system set up. The students received a VFS backpack with a water bottle and lots of other stuff inside. I soon found out why she was given the VFS umbrella—I've never seen so much rain in my life!

I was interested in what she was taking and she would let me know what she was up to in each term. Jenny explained to me that Term One was intensive for developing drawing and animation skills and basic art through life drawing. She told me she loved doing the character design and learning about film theory and the history of animation. Jenny told me some of the extra classes she took were Story Concept and Camera Technique. I remember her telling me in Term Two that there was more expansion on life drawing, and that it was a bit weird at first for her to see a person naked, especially a male. Jenny and I had a good laugh, because of her facial expressions when she talked to me about that.

Jenny felt very comfortable with her schooling, and would bring her life art home. There was so much more in the other terms and I could see Jenny was loving every minute of it. In Term Four, they started to learn all the components required to make their short films. I remember in Term Five, Jenny practically lived at the school, early mornings and late nights. She ate, breathed, and talked animation in her sleep. Term Six, she concentrated on the post-production of her short film along with other work. Jenny explained to me that with this Classical Animation Course, she learned the entire animation process from concept development to the short film she made. She said it included animation drawing techniques, storyboarding, layout, background, and character design. She loved working in traditional animation and enjoyed learning the Adobe® Flash® software. Jenny was happy to know that upon graduating she would get a copy of her animation project film, the Flash film, and a portfolio of her art and animation.

Jenny was in her element and couldn't get enough of it. Her passion and dedication were evident in her work. There were even a few occasions when she stayed at school overnight in order to meet a deadline. Jenny always liked to be on top or ahead of the game with her studies and first-year films.

Jenny and her classmates would take breaks in between classes to go eat, get some air, and socialize. I would take some of her group to film viewings or places they needed to go or get home from. They were a lovely group of young women and men. She was meeting some really nice people whose company she enjoyed, and vice versa. There were some Canadians, though the majority were from the United States, Japan, China, Mexico, Brazil, Spain, and elsewhere around the world. They would go out for suppers, movies, picnics, or meet at each other's places or the beach.

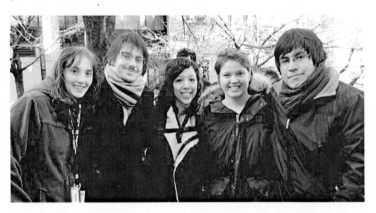

Jenny hangs out with her 2D Classical Animation friends: Jenny, Stefano, Caroline, Sol, and Omar.

On her birthday, they got her a *Nightmare before Christmas* cake, presents, and a musical birthday candle. Jenny was overwhelmed and thought it was so nice of them. They would all go to animation conventions and events together. They even took the skytrain to see a Roller Derby event in Richmond, as one of the student's wives was on a team. It was the first time Jenny had seen a Roller Derby in action.

It was so wonderful to see Jenny socializing and feeling part of a group. Her classmates called her the "cute, quiet one." She was shy; however, she did open up as time went on and got to know everybody. Jenny still found it hard to socialize and battled with the everlasting self-doubts: "Did I say it right?" "Did I answer right?" "I hope I didn't say anything that made them not like me!" But these doubts weren't nearly as debilitating.

After much hard work and long hours, giving it her usual one hundred and ten percent, Jenny graduated from the 2D Classical Animation course. VFS screened the students' films at the Graduation Ceremony. and each student was called up one by one to receive their diplomas. When Jenny's name was called, I cheered out for her and took pictures. I can't even describe the emotions and feelings going through me at this point. Time stood still once again as I watched her take her diploma and join the others up on stage. A proud moment for any parent, but considering the obstacles she had faced it was even more elating for me. We cheered the whole class after everyone had received their diplomas, and everyone sat down to screen the films.

All the films were really good. Jenny's were awesome; she's become quite the comedian—she had all of us laughing out loud. Her first film was called "Where's the Honey?" and it was about a mama and a baby bear who were trying to get to a bee's nest for honey. It had a great story, characters, music, and theme. Her second film, which I must say is my favourite, was called "Happy Birthday" and it was about a mother and her daughter celebrating the daughter's birthday. It evolved around the wicked birthday candle that wouldn't blow out. Her animation, storyline, the characters, the voice-over work, and the music were seriously well done. After it was finished everyone was cheering and clapping. I know that made her feel good about herself and who she is as an animator. I told her how funny her films were and that people really enjoyed them and she smiled to me, "They laughed, Mum."

When the ceremony was over, we went to a reception party where they had put out tons of food, desserts, and drinks. The class went up on stage opening bottles of champagne and cheering their triumph. Jenny held the glass but didn't drink much as she doesn't like the taste of alcohol.

This was another accomplishment—to see Jenny with her classmates having a good time—sitting with them and laughing, talking, mingling with them all. I sat and watched her converse and engage, being part of the group, being included. I know this meant a lot to her. They liked Jenny for who she is and that was a huge boost to her self-esteem. In saying this, I know at times she would still second-guess herself in social situations. Jenny never actually told her classmates about her autism or being special needs. She didn't want that to influence their opinions of her—she wanted them to know and like her for who she is now and has become. It was a fresh start with new people and she wanted as much as possible to put the autism behind her. I totally understood and respected her for this.

Once she graduated from the 2D Classical Animation program, she was accepted into the 3D Digital Character

Animation program. Although Jenny was incredibly excited to be accepted, she had the choice to start right away
in September or wait until January. We talked about her
options, and I suggested that it might be nice to take a little
break after all her hard work the past year, especially as she
had gone straight into VFS from high school. Jenny had
already decided to take a break, but had wanted to talk to
me about it. I thought she made a good decision.

From September to December, she had a chance to relax
and revisit the book she had written. Always in the back
of her mind, Jenny remembered what Mrs. Wallberg said
about getting her book published. We had so much going
on with the move and her schooling that this was the first
opportunity we had to find a publisher. We reached out to
a couple of publishers Mrs. Wallberg had given us; however, Jenny's book didn't fit into their genre or age group.
They did, however, love the chapters Jenny had sent them.

A lovely friend of mine, Bernadette Saquibal, sent me
an email about a publishing company that was inviting
writers to come to its open house event. Jenny and I went
and met some lovely people, including Julie Salisbury, the
founder of Influence Publishing. She was very interested
in Jenny's book but it didn't fit their genres at that time.
I explained Jenny's story and how I had been wanting to
write a book about her life. Julie looked at me intently and
said she had been wanting to find someone to do a story on
autism. She mentioned how sweet it would be to publish
our books together. We let Julie know that Jenny had one
more important year of animation school, but encouraged
Julie to contact us the following year as we would love to
get together with her again. I could tell Julie was keen on
the idea and looked forward to meeting us again. We put

the book on the back burner while Jenny prepared for another intense year of school.

During this time, we met with a couple of people from the "Youth Transition Program with Developmental Disabilities Association": Pierre Tardif and Peggy Liu. They came to our home and explained a program they offer that would help Jenny with her everyday life—enabling her to be more independent as opposed to relying on me. I would do anything for her, but I believe she needs to trust in herself and be able to do things on her own.

The big goals were communication, doing bank transactions by herself, going on a bus and subway by herself, and holding a conversation independently. Additionally, we wanted her to be able to order at a restaurant in an audible voice. They also worked on Jenny going to a grocery store and buying her own food, by making a shopping list, purchasing the items needed, and carrying them home independently.

Peggy and Jenny (with my help in setting up meetings) would go on outings to do things together. Over time, Jenny learned to use the buses and to order food in an audible voice. In time, when she visited the grocery store, she would go to the correct aisles for items and pick out brands she liked or preferred. She was able to pay and get the change and receipt independently. Jenny was also getting better at recalling information regarding bus routes and itineraries, and was able to choose her preferred route.

These coping skills were incredibly valuable, as they were transferable to when she was out with friends going to restaurants or riding the skytrain. Initially, Jenny and I would go to the bank together. At first she wanted me right by her side; but in time I needed to let her handle things by herself. Jenny has come along leaps and bounds with this and is now a bit more comfortable and secure in herself and her daily activities. I appreciate all that Peggy did with Jenny and the times they spent together. Jenny really liked Peggy and felt comfortable with her and trusted her, as did I. Jenny had matured so much in that year. At times, she falls back and gets nervous, and she still lives at home with us, but she has to look after a lot of her own things and pays rent.

January 2013 arrived and it was time for Jenny to go to the orientation session for the 3D Digital Character Animation program. She was so happy to be back and looking forward to diving into this year as well. A couple of her fellow students from Classical Animation were in this class, which made her happy; however the majority were new students from all over the world. She made some great friends from this class, and they did a lot of things together. From what I saw in her second year at VFS, she had to work even harder and was expected to do a lot more in a shorter period of time. Once again, she would be there early mornings, late evenings, every weekend, and sometimes overnight. This was a heavy class schedule. There was the odd day she would be emotional and frustrated, but they were few and far between considering all that was asked of her in this course. She put every inch of herself into classes and her film for graduation.

Even though Jenny had a heavy workload, I was happy to see her get out for suppers, movies, picnics, and other social gatherings. She would join her classmates in attending animation events, including the Fan Expo Vancouver—fascinating to animators. It was great to see how they were there for one another, celebrating each other's birthdays with cards, cakes, and outings. Between school, work, and finances, they did as much as they possibly could to keep sane while in the course.

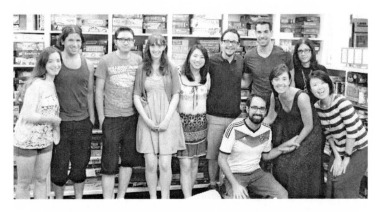

Jenny is out for an evening with her 3D Digital Character Animation friends

Jenny explained to me that this course was for experienced classical animators and that she would broaden her animation skills by going through cinematic storytelling skills, classical animation techniques, and digital operating environments. She was looking forward to developing a short film to showcase her abilities.

One of the highlights while she was in this course happened outside school. I took Jenny to Fan Expo Vancouver at the Convention Centre, as Sean Astin was going to be there. She really liked him in *The Goonies*, but more so, she is a *Teenage Mutant Ninja Turtles* fan, and he is the voice of Raphael in the new *Turtles* series. She had drawn a picture of Sean as Raphael and wanted to give it to him.

While we were in line and getting closer to him, she was so nervous that she whispered to me, "I feel sick to my stomach and I might throw up." We had waited so long and she was then one person away, so I said, "Look, just breathe, take my hand and, if you feel sick, I have a bag you can puke in." I couldn't believe I even said that but I knew if we dropped out of line she would be even more upset and sick. I got her to take deep breaths and let loose, which she did. She hung in there and—boom—she was in front of him.

Sean was very nice to her and was really impressed with her drawing of Raphael. He signed it for her and said to hang it up in her room. Sean said to Jenny how much he loved her full name of Jenny Story and that it is an awesome name for an animator to have, and then took a picture with her. As we walked away she was feeling much better and the colour started returning to her cheeks. She thanked me for having her stay in line so that she could meet him.

The six months for this course went by quickly and she made it through. It was graduation time again for Jenny as she had passed and is now a Professional 3D Digital Character Animator. They showed a Class Grad Video at the graduation ceremony, and it was great to see Jenny and her classmates enjoying their school time. Once again they showed everyone's films after the certificates were issued. Jenny's film was called "Alienated," and it was so sweet. It was about a lonely alien who, when he cried, had waterfalls of water pouring out of his eyes. Hilarious! Everyone was killing themselves laughing. She is a very talented animator. The amount of time, work, and patience a person needs for this is unreal. I give Jenny and all of them so much credit for their love of this field of work, and how it entertains the world.

Chapter Fourteen

Full Circle

As of today, we are still living in Vancouver and Jenny has met a lot of people and made lovely friends within her animation circles. Of course, Vernon will always be a special city to us in so many ways and "home" in our hearts—we cherish so many people there.

It is hard to believe we have been here for over three years already and Jenny has graduated, and is now a professional animator. I respect her hard work and dedication to all she takes on, and admire the non-stop commitment she displayed in both of the animation courses she took at VFS. Jenny was constantly drawing when she was a child, and I remember thinking her hand would fall off or stop working, she drew so much. I thought drawing was very therapeutic for her in handling all she was going through. I was always in awe of her art work. Jenny's imagination shone through her stories and characters. She was in her element drawing, and all that has happened to her was meant to be. Jenny has closets crammed with books full of her stories and drawings.

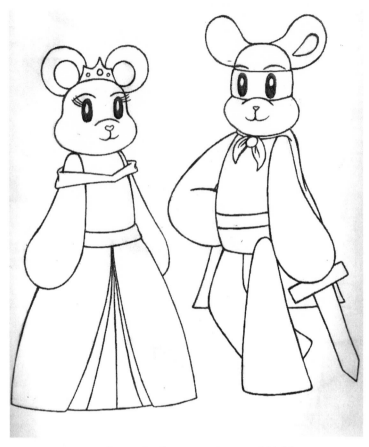

Two of Jenny's Characters, Rosa and Teddy

When Jenny graduated from Vancouver Film School, she worked on her resume and cover letter, and incorporated her animation films and drawings into a website (jennystory.ca). She was looking forward to getting on board with an animation studio; however, something else was put in front of her: the book she had started back in high school.

Jenny told me this story came from a dream she had—that the ideas just started flooding her mind and she began writing them down and crafting them into a story. At this point, we received a call-back email from Influence Publishing, inviting us to their publishing event. There, we spoke to Julie again and learned even more about the company and what was involved with publishing through them. It turned out the company had ventured into different genres of books, which was promising for Jenny and her novel. Julie and her staff were so professional yet personable when answering our questions.

We received a folder of materials describing Influence and what the publishing process entails. I was so impressed with this folder; it was informative and it showed the genuine dedication and care the company has for its authors. To Jenny and me, deciding to publish with Influence was a no-brainer.

Jenny and I left the event feeling we had found the right publishing company. I looked at her and asked, "Are you ready for another adventure and another dream of yours to come true?"

She smiled and was both excited and nervous simultaneously. We were both in a bit of a haze, because of what was happening. It was as if we had caught another rainbow, another pot of gold for Jenny. Julie and the company were definitely interested and, in talking with them, Jenny and I decided we would both take part in their writing workshop. We wanted them to get to know who we are, and to feel out our books—to explore the potential of their being published. We are forever grateful to Bernadette for giving us the information about Influence so we could check them out.

I had a conversation with Jenny about me writing a book about her. I wanted to make sure she would be okay with it as I would be exposing her life to the public. I wanted to respect her privacy and see what her feelings were on my writing about who she is and the trials and tribulations she has endured. If she didn't want me to, I would have totally understood and not done it. However, Jenny's answer revealed once again what a caring, kind, and genuine young woman she is. She said to me, "Mum, I don't mind you writing this book about me. If it can help a family or their child with autism or special needs, then your book is a good thing and my story will be beneficial."

That really hit me hard when she said this as I truly feel the same way. I wanted to write this book to help parents, autistic children, and autistic individuals. I wanted to show what one has to do to get help, find support, and battle that uphill climb to get every resource we possibly can. To never look back, to never give up—even when we feel we are hitting our heads against a brick wall. We must always be that solid rock and foundation for our children and ourselves. I hope in your reading my book and seeing how Jenny's life turned around, you can see that anything is possible, and you too can follow that yellow brick road to a bright and successful future. I want her story and Jenny as an individual to offer a ray of hope and sunshine to everyone.

Jenny and I signed up for Influence Publishing's InspireABook weekend intensive mastermind workshop. We were given pre-workshop worksheets and spent ample time answering the questions specifically to enhance the purpose of our books.

Julie said, "You have given yourself a gift of this weekend's workshop, so come prepared to dedicate the whole weekend to 'eat and breathe your book.' Be sure to come with lots of energy." Jenny and I were game for it all and dedicated the weekend to the workshop.

We enjoyed listening to Julie and Lyda as they were both so knowledgeable in the book business and the art of writing. They wanted our experience to be wonderful and enjoyable in addition to us learning the ins and outs of the publishing industry. At one point over the weekend, Julie wanted us all to get to know about each other's books. It was overwhelming and wonderful to see Jenny talk about her book in front of everyone, and discuss the "mind map" she'd prepared to show the storyline of her novel. I knew she was nervous but she stuck it out and did an excellent job with her explanations and conversing with other people. Afterwards, she said she had been so anxious that she felt she hadn't done so well—but I told her she had done very well, and that everyone else thought so too.

Julie Salisbury gave us contract information documents as she felt confident in both our books and wanted to sign us on. We had to fill out proposal forms once we completed the workshop; publishing our books was subject to Influence's approval.

It was a highly interactive two days for us both, and Jenny and I met some lovely people with whom we stay in touch. We both worked on our books and it was very inspiring and a lot of fun as well. We were so happy and thrilled when Jenny's book was approved.

We were also lucky to listen, meet, and talk with Bennett R. Coles who is a prize-winning fantasy novel writer. Jenny was excited to meet him as this is right up her alley, and he was excited about Jenny's book and wanted to read it. This meant a lot to Jenny and we talked about it all the way home. Coles read her book and really enjoyed it; he suggested that she could write two follow-up books and make the three a trilogy.

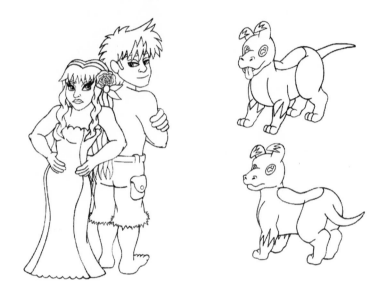

Characters from Jenny's novel, *Dysnomia*

She is now a professional animator and an author, all at twenty-one years old. I remember Julie saying Jenny is the youngest person to have done their workshop and how mature she is. She is so humble about these huge accomplishments. Her personality has not changed. She has always been the most honest, sincere, and genuine young lady you could ever meet. She is a joy and makes this world a better place.

Jenny and I drove to Influence Publishing's office on March 6, 2014 and we met up with Julie Salisbury, Gulnar Patel, and Alina Wilson. Jenny and I both signed our publishing agreement contracts. We took pictures together with the bouquet of flowers and a card we gave Julie to thank her for signing us on. It was a very exciting day and we went out for supper to celebrate; another treasured memory for Jenny and me. We have been back and forth a few times for meetings and discussions and going through all the guidelines for our books. Gulnar, Alina, and Julie have all been wonderful with every aspect of publishing our books. Dreams come true—work hard and believe in yourself and have the drive to make it happen.

This past year, Jenny has been putting all her energy and hard work into her book with writing, editing, marketing, and all the last-minute details. Jenny really dug deep during the editing process, as it was a lot of work. Once again, she was game for the challenge. She is working on her own illustrations for the book as well, which is really exciting. In July, she had her author photo taken. We actually did this together for both our books and we had so much fun. I couldn't have wished for a better bonding moment between a mother and a daughter. It will be so special to go out together to do book signings, meeting people, and talking to them about our books. It will be a good experience for Jenny discussing her work with strangers. She has told me that she will be very nervous; however, I have assured her I will be right by her side. I'm so excited for people to meet and talk with Jenny when they see this is the young lady who my book is about. I feel this will be such a unique experience for the public to share with both of us. We look forward to meeting everyone.

Jenny has come so far and has so much more to look forward to in her life. Her future will be bright and shining. She already has a sequel to her book in her head and will start getting it on paper after the first book is all done. She is also planning on returning to animation by getting back into producing her own short films, and has been asked to work on a short film for a production company. Who knows what will come up next? Feature films and an animated TV series of her books? Time will tell. She will keep reaching for the stars like she has been doing—the sky's the limit.

There is no telling what the future holds for Jenny, but if it is anything like what has been happening for her so far, buckle up, as we are in for a fantastic ride with her, and she richly deserves all that comes her way.

What a privilege it has been to go on this journey and relive my daughter's life. It has brought back so much that I remember vividly and there are moments in writing that have jogged events in my brain that I had long forgotten. Some of the memories have been so tough to write about and they made me cry. And there are beautiful outstanding memories that put such a huge grin on my face and warmed my heart. It has been a long, unique adventure from when Jenny was diagnosed and a series of ups and downs, laughs and tears. To watch Jenny unfold right in front of my eyes and to see her eventually get to know herself, believe in herself, and be confident in herself—in her intelligence, talent, and looks—has been such a privilege. She also learned to become assertive and stick up for herself.

Jenny is still quiet and shy. Her conversation and socialization has come along from what it was and it's wonderful to see her start conversations and interact. I know she can have some issues, but she deals with them very well and she and I always have a heart-to-heart to settle her issues. I see at times when she is nervous or having trouble with conversation or answering. It is subtle, yet I see the anguish and tension going through her and her eyes welling up. My heart goes out to her at these times and I will ease in to help her out in certain situations, which I attempt to do in a non-invasive way so as not to embarrass her or reveal how she is feeling at the moment. She has told me it is still hard at times. Yet I know Jenny wants to get out there and socialize and be part of the group. She has actually even initiated some of the outings with her friends. That is a huge leap for her. It fills my heart with joy when things like this happen. She will come home and tell me what a great time she has had and that she is going out again as they are doing something else. Jenny will always have some aspects of autism and special needs for the rest of her life. However, she has conquered a lot of it as well, which truly evolved from—number one—Jenny's hard work and perseverance; and number two—from the work put in by myself, her family, and all those who supported her. Jenny is truly a walking miracle.

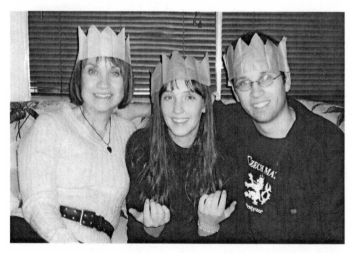

Jenny sits with her auntie Vicki and cousin Paul at Christmas.

What Others Shared: Vicki Brown

When my sister Vicki was visiting last year, she commented and said, "It is a privilege watching Jenny grow into a beautiful and talented young person who has developed her artistic gifts through hard work and determination. Some artwork from her childhood is still on my walls at home. Jenny may appear to be timid to those who do not know her but she is a confident, bright, and caring person whose attractive appearance is topped off with a gorgeous smile."

Jenny certainly is a role model for us all because of all she has been through. She shows every single one of us that we can do anything we put our minds to if we work hard and believe in ourselves no matter what obstacles lie in front of us. She kept trooping, kept climbing, was patient and calm, and dealt with adversity. She is kind to others, because of her loving, caring nature. I love my daughter's spirit and her determination—her hard-work ethic. The exposure of all this with her growing up in front of me has been an eye-opening and a once-in-a-lifetime experience. It has been a transformation for me and our entire family, friends and professionals who know and have been around Jenny. She is an example of true heroism with her autism and special needs journey. Jenny has taken life by the reins and pulled it all in, achieving her goals and dreams. I always visualize her life as though she has climbed to the peak of the mountain, with her now being an animator and a writer. She has broken down many a barrier and brick wall that was put in front of her in order to reach those peaks.

She is the epitome of what a person does against all odds as she tackles and defeats anything standing in her way.

I am so happy for my daughter and of course very proud of her and all she has done. To have Jenny as my daughter is a true blessing and I treasure her and the relationship we have as mother and daughter. I enjoy every minute with her; she makes me laugh so hard and vice versa. We really are the best of friends. Even with the issues at hand and the seriousness of facing her autism and special needs, we have had wonderful times and have an abundant chest full of memories that we are constantly adding to.

Epilogue

Memories From Past to Present

I include this with heartfelt love to show my readers the fun and enjoyable times we had as a family. In between all the hard work there were many happy times. These were a big help with Jenny's zeal for life.

I mentioned in a previous chapter how Jenny and I went to many of the beaches in the Okanagan area, as we were both passionate about going to the beach and swimming. It was always such a beautiful bonding time for us to share together. Jenny was like a dolphin. She loved the water slides, especially the tubes. We would also go to our local pools and go swimming, play on the rafts, jump off the rope, throw the balls back and forth. We wondered if she might be a competitive swimmer as she got older; she was strong and I could see her being a contender. However, that did not appeal to her professionally.

On many a day you would find me and Jenny playing a game of badminton outside in the backyard. Then as she got older we tried tennis. Croquet was also something we set up and had a lot of fun playing. Jenny was competitive and she was really good at any game she took on. I am the same.

Jenny and I also loved going to the local fairs like the Interior Provincial Exhibition in Armstrong. We went every year starting from when she was a little girl. She loved the rides, going to the events, and especially seeing all the animals—like the rabbits, goats, and cows. Jenny loves animals and she actually considered becoming a veterinarian. She doesn't like to see animals hurting, and is so caring and gentle toward them. When she got older, we also took in the Pacific National Exhibition in Vancouver, and since we moved here we have gone nearly every year. Last year they had an Animation Building, which thrilled her, and she took us around describing everything to us and explaining what different displays meant. It made us so happy to see the zeal she felt for it all, and we were impressed that she knew all of the animators they had biographies on, both young and old. We actually couldn't get her out of there as she didn't want to miss a single thing on display.

Because of her love for animals, I would take her to Davison Orchards and Chickadee Ridge Miniatures as they held ongoing events. She loved the horse wagon rides and their barn dances, the children's entertainment and crafts. She fell in love with the pot-bellied pig at Chickadee Ridge and wanted to take him home. That didn't happen, but we went back many times so she could see him. Jenny would take every animal home if she could. I remember our first visit to the Falkland Rodeo. Jenny was young, around four or five years old, and we were watching the rodeo when the event for calf roping began. She of course had never seen this before, and when they started roping the little calf she got very upset, and stood up screaming, "Stop, don't do that." We had to leave as she was crying and getting mad. I felt bad for her and we had a good, long hugging session. Needless to say, there was no more calf roping for Jenny, and I can understand why she felt that way.

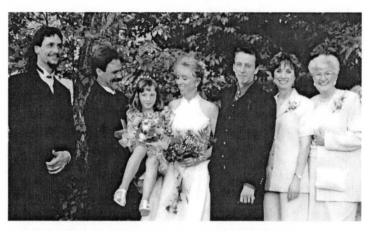

Our family poses outside the church on our wedding day: John (Travis's brother), Travis, Jenny, me, Chris, my sister Vicki, and my mother, Vera.

When Travis and I were married on July 10, 1999, Jenny was our flower girl and Chris took me up the aisle. It was very emotional for me to watch them both be an integral and big part of our wedding. Jenny was only six years old and she did such a good job in her role. She was patient and quiet while she stood up front with us during the whole ceremony and for the signing of the register book. However, as time went on for the picture taking, she became tired and bored with it all. Jenny kept resting on Travis's and my shoulders, and wanting to be held. At one point, she found a swing set on the church grounds and had fun swinging. There was a funny moment with Jenny at our reception after we had eaten the main course, because she kept asking to go home; but when they brought out the cake and ice cream, she came back to life very quickly. The look on her face was priceless. We actually have kept her bouquet—a beautiful memory.

One of Jenny's favourite TV shows when she was in Grade 6—*Lizzie Maguire*—featured Hilary Duff—she liked Duff's music and had all her CDs. So I surprised Jenny and bought us tickets to see Duff in concert in Vancouver. That was a highlight for Jenny and one she still remembers. I know Jenny wasn't into dancing and singing herself at that time; however, she was up dancing and singing with me that night, and we had a great mother/daughter weekend. I also surprised her with a road trip to Seattle in 2011 to go and see the stage production of *Wicked*, which she loved. Jenny and I had a great time. We also enjoyed going to the stage production of *Beauty and the Beast* in Vancouver in 2012.

We had many a trip over the years to the Vancouver Aquarium as Jenny's favourite was the orca whale and she loved the *Free Willy* movies. She was actually obsessed with them and had a ton of Orca stuffies, pictures, posters, PJs, blankets, pillows, clothes, and books. Anything you could get with an orca on it or about it, she had it. In 2008, we went to Victoria for a holiday; the highlight of the vacation was whale watching. To see the look on Jenny's face when we were lucky enough to have a pod come close by us was heaven. I will never forget the look on her face and the awe she had for the orcas. She also liked Science World in Vancouver as she was keen on learning how things worked.

We took trips out of town too, visiting places like West Edmonton Mall, and the following year we drove out to the

Prairies where I had been born in Manitoba. The landscape was quite a shock for Jenny, as she was raised in Vernon and had never seen the flatness of the prairies before. She kept asking where the mountains were, but all we could show her were a few hills. She loved the Winnipeg Zoo and when we were in Regina she loved the museum with the dinosaurs. We visited Drumheller when she was in her young teens, and she thoroughly enjoyed their dinosaur museum and exhibits.

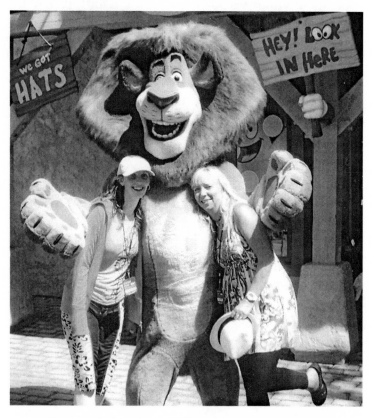

Jenny and I have fun with "Alex" from *Madagascar* at Universal Studios.

Our biggest trip was going to Disneyland, California Adventure Park, Universal Studios, San Diego Zoo, and SeaWorld San Diego. Travis, Jenny, and I drove down there from Vernon in July 2010, and I have never seen Jenny so excited. She was looking forward to being in Disneyland and also to see all the animation as well. I had been wanting to go there myself since I was five, and Jenny had always wanted to go. When we walked through the gates at Disneyland, we all turned into ten year olds! We took in everything we possibly could, and the highlight for Jenny was going to the Animation Studio in the California Adventure Park, where she got to draw, do a voice over, and see which animation character she would be, which for her was Jane from the *Tarzan* movie. Most of all she liked learning to draw with the Disneyland animator; he loved her work, which made her happy and even more interested in becoming an animator.

We all had a very interesting surprise on our second night in Disneyland. We had just finished eating and Travis went to the washroom. When he came back he said, "There is someone here who knows you," and I said, "What?" I didn't know anyone who was going to be there. So we walked over to see this person and—what a lovely surprise—it was Justin Dorval, my son's good friend from his youth—the one I mentioned earlier in the book who rescued me and helped take Jenny home from the park when she was having a fit. I mean what are the odds?

One of Jenny's favourite rides was at Universal Studios—it was the Jurassic Park Ride, due to her love of dinosaurs and the *Jurassic Park* movies.

However, the most treasured moments for me are not the big outings or going far away, but the precious memories of being at home with Jenny. For example, enjoying playing board games together, doing puzzles, and colouring. We loved to go and rent a movie or game and enjoy it with a bowl of popcorn; baking in the kitchen and watching her lick the spoon; having her friends over for sleepovers or birthday parties and taking them bowling or tobogganing; and playing pin the tail on the donkey and hitting the Piñatas.

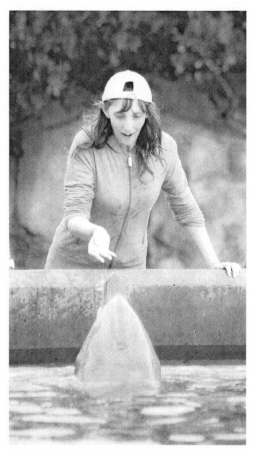

A young dolphin really takes to Jenny at SeaWorld San Diego.

One thing that Jenny and I have always done since she was a little girl and still do to this day when we are both home together at night is to have a hot drink together. Jenny has her hot chocolate and I have my tea. It is our special bonding time and we talk about what has gone on during our day or what is on our minds. Bringing Jenny into this world and sharing so many wonderful moments with her is a blessing and an honour, and I am proud to be her mother. I thank Jenny for being such a wonderful daughter and person, and for enriching my life. I will always be her rock, her listening ear, her security and—most of all—her number one cheerleader in all she does.

I must mention the importance of working with a close knit team for your child and family, as I had with our Dream Team and our Respite Angels, so as not to diminish all the hard efforts and work that has been done for Jenny. This is far from an overnight job. This is a long journey, not only for us, but for Jenny herself to get where she is today. It is integral to have a loving, caring, devoted, professional, and personable group of people working for you and your child. I thank God every day for this wonderful group of people who came into our lives, who devoted every minute of their time to Jenny, which in turn helped to develop the intelligent, talented, and beautiful young woman she is today.

To all readers, especially autistic families and autistic individuals, look for the light at the end of the dark tunnel. Reach out to that rainbow of colours and at the end grab that pot of gold that is yours to enjoy. Believe in yourselves and do anything you want or dream of. Go for it and trust in Jenny's story to inspire your own story. She and I believe in you and your families.

Remember that being autistic and having special needs (well, I always say "normal with special needs") is not a life sentence. It is eye opening to your soul and being. Use your autism and special needs in a positive avenue to reach for the stars. Shine bright, fly high, and enjoy your life. In sharing Jenny's life with the public our hope is that it shines a bright light and an adventurous avenue for others with autism and special needs so their lives can be as rewarding. I know it is Jenny's and my wish for this book to reach others.

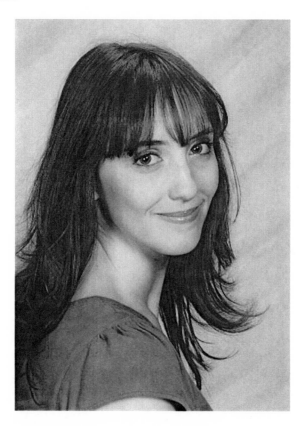

Appendix A

Son-Rise Program

Barry Neil and Samahria Kaufman created The Son-Rise Program® and the Autism Treatment Center of America® after successfully reaching their little boy Raun, a child who was "diagnosed as severely and incurably autistic" (www.AutismTreatment.org).

When I found out the Kaufmans had written a book on their successful method, I got it and read feverishly to the end; I couldn't put it down. I found the stories at the end of the book extremely interesting: other parents were talking about the scenarios with their own autistic children. One thing they mentioned was their children being severely sick after having a vaccination. Their children had the same type of physical reactions and illness and, most importantly, the same mental changes regarding speech, play, talking, and socializing as had my Jenny. I knew this couple had discovered something that worked and I wanted to take Jenny to Sheffield to take part in The Son-Rise Program® at the Autism Centre of America® right away.

When I read and saw all the wonderful positive reports of children and their families, it was a godsend.

However, I was a single mum, working full time and taking care of my son and my daughter; it was not something I could afford. So I did the next best thing. I got their books, manuals, and tapes, and I shared them with Brer Rabbit Day Care, North Okanagan Neurological Society and, of course, with the Speech and Play Therapist. We modelled their techniques and methods, which were eye openers to us in reaching out to Jenny.

I was overwhelmed, enlightened, relieved, and put at ease to read parents' letters in The Son-Rise Program® manuals. These were people from all over the world, each going through their own trial and tribulations; some of the parents were quite depressed. I remember one woman wrote that her doctor told her that her daughter might never have friends or a sense of humour and only engage in isolated activities for the rest of her life. Imagine how that woman was feeling. It was like telling her that her child's future is completely futile.

It hit me hard as I felt her pain; it was similar to what they had told me would be Jenny's life. I cannot say I got depressed though and I never went on medication. The poor diagnosis made me assertive, like a mother lion protecting and being there for her cub. I felt emotional pain for my daughter and her being withdrawn always broke my heart, but it made me fight even harder.

Some people find this experience in their life overwhelming. They ask why they and their child are so unlucky. I am thankful that I was able to turn it into a positive insight in my life and to appreciate who and what my child is.

It reminds me of a moment one day when I was standing

in a line-up in Shoppers Drug Mart. A woman standing in front of me was talking to the cashier about her autistic child and what a burden he was, which made her so mad and her life so difficult. I mean I was in shock, stunned, and horrified to hear that. I felt so much for that boy and wanted to say something, in a kind manner. But the mother stomped off in a huff. Caring for an autistic child is a non-stop twenty-four-hour-a-day commitment, as you have to be there one hundred and ten percent—and then some—for your child's mental and physical well-being. For me, Jenny is my little girl and a precious gift.

This reminds me of what the Kaufmans say to people who are overwhelmed with their special child: "They are not a curse, but a gift … a gift which challenges us to respond with enormous energy, dedication and love. Finding a way to help that child, to be there in the most loving, supporting and facilitating way possible. Such a process is a daily moment to moment treasure for us all."

Oh, my goodness. This hit my heart and my very soul; it is how I feel in being and working with Jenny—so eloquently put. I always remember the moment I read this and how it struck me. I mean, as a parent, we are looking out for our child's best interests. We are the most powerful advocates and the most dedicated, useful, and loving resource they have. Giving this love and lifetime interest in your child brings out the very best in them and yourself.

Samahria Kaufman stated, "As long as a child is alive, there is hope!"

When the doctor told me everything that Jenny would be unable to do, they basically put her in a corner. What the doctor did to me was the exact same thing the Kaufmans went through with Raun. It is like closing a door on your child and never letting them in. One should be made hopeful and given positive energy and optimism. We always have to remember that doctors are not gods and what they predict does not say how things will be. Raun and Jenny are wonderful examples of this.

The Kaufmans encourage parents of autistic children to allow their child to be his or her own teacher, as well as the parents' teacher. They encourage parents to disallow their children to be judged or labelled because of their behaviour, as they are doing the best they can with what they have.

I remember when Jenny would act up in public and people would give us both awful, disgusted looks and make mean comments. I was always having to repeat myself and explain. Then I finally stopped doing that as my little girl was truly a sweetheart and she was handling the situation as best she could. She could not help it: she had autism, and that is how she reacted to the situation in front of her. If she could have handled it better, if she could have talked or conversed or interacted she would have. How very frustrating it must have been for her; I cannot possibly imagine. We had to enter and understand her world and encourage a loving, trusting bond to grow.

Here are some final words from the Kaufmans and The Son-Rise Program® that have stuck close to me. They said that, when asked, "What is autism?" they would explain that it is a complex development disability that appears usually around the first three years of age. It was more common in boys than in girls, back then. It is a development disability that has challenges in language, communication, emotions, cognition, behaviour, fine and gross motor skills, and social interaction. This is the absolute pinpoint of the diagnosis of autism with Jenny. They went on to say that autistic children engage in repetitive activities, stereotyped movements, resistance to environmental change, and difficulties with communication and sensory experiences. Jenny followed suit in those areas as well.

What pierced my heart, soul, and mind is what was said next, what The Son-Rise Program® proclaims: "Autism does not have to be a Life Sentence!"

That statement is so powerful and meaningful that every parent should etch it inside their heads. That hit me like a bolt of lightning and it was my intent to inspire hope for Jenny, to help her achieve her dreams so that she could fulfill her potential and take meaningful action in whatever she wanted to do. Throughout Jenny's life, I have always been consistently positive and optimistic for her present and future. That became life-affirming for her as she grew up and improved every day. She started to believe in herself and reach goals that I told her she could most definitely do where others told her she could not.

Follow those dreams, break through those barriers. Life with autism is not a dark tunnel; it is a bright ray of sunshine, happiness, and fulfillment. It is there to be grabbed and, for what an autistic child goes through, it is justly deserved.

Appendix B

Vaccines

The haunting change in Jenny after she got sick as a baby immediately following her twelve-month vaccination shot left me desperately seeking out any potential explanation. It was such a shock to the system to see her entire personality do a complete 180° turn. One day, she was saying words, engaging in eye contact, reacting, and playing with her peers—she was a little entertainer. I used to say she was a mini-me. I saw such a thriving little girl who was developing normally with no concerns at all. The next day, she had ceased communicating, would not make eye contact, wouldn't socialize, and flew into fits, hurting herself. It was so distressing and unexplainable, and I just kept praying I would wake up from the nightmare and Jenny would be back to herself.

Was this a coincidence? Had she had a reaction to one of the ingredients in the vaccine? No one could tell me what happened. No medical professional could give me an answer. I needed to know what had happened to my little girl.

I felt so helpless—how could I protect her from such an invisible threat? I couldn't shake the suspicion that the vaccine might have been to blame; it kept going over and over in my mind. Had it caused an allergic reaction, causing her to become extremely sick, and that's why we just about lost her? After researching the topic, I discovered other parents had children who had experienced the same type of reaction, and they too lost the child they knew before.

Rest assured I am NOT recommending parents avoid vaccinating their children, nor do I think it is wrong to do so. I DO, however, strongly believe that babies and young children should have a blood test or allergy test beforehand, to ensure they won't react to any of the substances in the vaccine. Or perhaps it would be safer to inject the substances separately, rather than all at once. So many children don't react to inoculation beyond a little fever or sluggishness, but there are those who react violently and, consequently, I believe we should be taking an extra step to ensure a child can tolerate the vaccine before it is administered. I say this with love and respect for every child and their parents.

I read an article entitled "The Case Against Immunizations," written by Richard Moskowitz, M.D., and published in the *Journal of the American Institute of Homeopathy* (76:7, March 1983). Dr. Moskowitz had noted that back in June 1978 a nine-month-old girl was brought in to see him with a fever of 105° Fahrenheit. This was the second time it had happened for this child and both occasions were after her vaccines. It was also noted that she had an extremely high white blood cell count. When he looked at the slide of her blood sample, he recognized she had symptoms of pertussis (*aka* whooping cough). Since

1978, he had seen other cases of children who reacted to vaccines with high fevers and then chronic complaints from the parents of irritability, tantrums, and many ear infections. The children physically and mentally changed from their former selves.

Jenny's white blood count was also high and I recall her having ear infections after that.

Dr. Suzanne Humphries M.D., a practising kidney physician, commented that the vaccine industry isn't giving people both sides of the story, and that parents need to inform themselves before subjecting their children to vaccines that could potentially cause serious harm or death. She has had patients with kidney issues she feels were caused by vaccines. She says that inventors of vaccines have chosen a belief system in which infants are born with inadequate immune systems, which, therefore, require being vaccinated. Suzanne says a doctor doesn't know how to take care of an immune system, because a doctor was never taught about it in school. She says we have ended up with a whole society not knowing how an immune system works or how to take care of it.

Dr. Sherri J. Tenpenny, a doctor of neuromuscular skeletal medicine and author of the book, *Saying No to Vaccines*, talks about the lack of safety studies conducted on vaccines, and whether or not they are effective.

In the *USA Today*'s Health and Behavior News Section, on March 2, 2010, Carla K. Johnson wrote an article entitled "Though unproven, 1 in 4 parents believe vaccines cause autism." In this same article, Dr. Melinda Wharton, M.D., M.P.H. of the US Centers for Disease Control and Prevention said if we don't vaccinate, diseases will come back. Some doctors are taking a tough stand, asking vaccine-refusing parents to find another doctor, and calling them selfish.

Christine Vara's article, "Doctors Take a Stand for Immunizations" on September 2, 2011 (on shotofprevention.com) describes a segment of the *Today Show* that aired on September 1, 2011. The show featured National Broadcasting Company's Chief Medical Editor, Dr. Nancy Snyderman, exploring whether doctors should ban children who are not vaccinated. Christine also spoke with Dr. Scott Goldstein M.D., F.A.A.P. of Northwestern Children's Practice in Chicago; this pediatrician takes a very active approach regarding immunization education. He pointed out that the US Centers for Disease Control and Prevention and the American Academy of Pediatrics set the safest and most effective childhood vaccination schedule.

Other doctors are very concerned that the mercury in the vaccine preservative thimerosal would cause speech delays, learning disabilities, and neurological disorders in children. Many of them express their concerns on the website Vaccines Uncensored (vaccinesuncensored.org).

Also of interest is that if one could read a vaccine package before allowing the vaccine to be given to your child, you would read about the risks and side effects, one of which is autism.

I talked about a child getting a blood test or allergy test to see if they react to what substances are in the vaccines. According to the FDA's fact sheets, vaccines are brimming with toxins, dozens of chemicals, heavy metals, and allergens. And numerous objectionable ingredients such as monkey kidney and aborted fetal tissue. I did find out that mercury is in them, as is aluminum. There are antibiotics in them that aren't even approved for uninfected children, like Polymyxin B sulfate-trimethoprim (*aka* Polytrim), for example.

A huge debate over the safety and efficacy of vaccinations is raging in the Western world. I find it mind blowing. The sad part is that we are gambling with our children's lives and health, and as parents we are trying to protect them. I personally was fortunate to have a pediatrician who saw and understood Jenny's behaviour. I believe parents should be better informed about what is in the vaccines to make sure it won't cause a reaction for their child and make them sick. The nurse told me, "Your child may get a bit of a fever or redness around the area of the shot."

I didn't know that the vaccine package listed side effects. I also felt shunned by people when I said I would not vaccinate Jenny again. I was doing it out of love, because of how she had reacted and that reaction had affected her—otherwise she would have received her shots like my son did; he was fine. Each individual reacts differently and each individual's body is unique.

In meeting with other parents of autistic children, I was curious to know the beginnings and how it came to be for them. It was uncanny. I would actually get goose bumps as the ones I talked to had the same occurrence as ours. Their children got terribly ill after their vaccine—with high temperatures, vomiting, and diarrhea; becoming dehydrated and lethargic. The child they once knew was also gone, shut down, and living in their own world. It's not just a coincidence, at least in all of our scenarios.

Each parent must do what they feel is the right thing for their child when it comes to vaccinations. It is your right and your personal viewpoint that must be accepted. Going through what I did with Jenny, I personally know that I absolutely made the right choice to not have Jenny vaccinated after the twelve-month shot. She has been a healthy child and is very rarely sick with colds, flus, or "things going around." I know that all her friends since she was little were vaccinated and some of them were constantly sick and caught everything that came around. Whether it was because Jenny wasn't vaccinated any further or because she is just a really healthy girl, the decision not to vaccinate her again worked out positively for her.

Author Biography

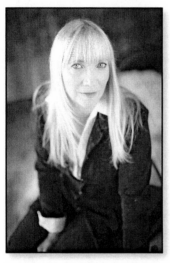

Janet Walmsley is a born-and-raised Manitoban who has lived in Vernon, British Columbia; Yellowknife, Northwest Territories; and Germany; she now lives in Vancouver, B.C. Along with being a mother, Janet has an active career in acting and singing; her theatre career spans well over a decade, while her comedic work in film, TV, and commercials has produced such nominations as the Annual Indie Awards in Los Angeles and the Leo Awards in Vancouver.

Janet is a mother of two: her son Christopher lives in Australia with his wife Ally; and her daughter Jenny lives in Vancouver with Janet and her husband Travis.

When her daughter Jenny was first diagnosed with autism, Janet went on a mission to support Jenny and autism awareness. Janet worked tirelessly alongside health professionals to provide every opportunity and avenue for her daughter, including fulfilling Jenny's dream to be an animator. In being Jenny's rock, Janet attended autism and special needs workshops, endlessly researched medical reports and articles, and talked with medical profession- als about autism. Janet attended all Jenny's appointments and ingested all that was said and done with Jenny so she could carry out the same activities at home. Travelling to talk to other families affected by autism, Janet researched and spoke to organizations to further her knowledge about caring for her daughter.

To learn more about Janet Walmsley, please visit:

Twitter
@janetwalmsley2

Linkedin
Janet Walmsley

Facebook
Personal Page: Janet Rollings Walmsley
Actor Page: J G Walmsley Vancouver Actor
Writer Page: Janet Walmsley & Jenny Story

If you want to get on the path to becoming a published author with Influence Publishing please go to www.InfluencePublishing.com

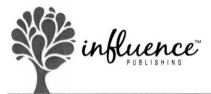

Inspiring books that influence change

More information on our other titles and how to submit your own proposal can be found at www.InfluencePublishing.com

CPSIA information can be obtained at www.ICGtesting.com
Printed in the USA
LVOW07s0823120515

438081LV00005B/135/P